# Multidisciplinary Perspectives on Aging

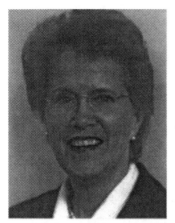

**Lynn M. Tepper, MA, MS, EdM, EdD,** is Associate Clinical Professor at Columbia University, and Director of the Institute of Gerontology at Mercy College. She has published extensively in the areas of family relationships in later life, counseling older people, service learning, long term care, and tobacco cessation in later life. Dr. Tepper has been awarded research funding from the National Institutes of Health, the National Institute on Aging, the National Institute for General Medical Sciences, and the U.S. Department of Education, supporting projects which focus on gerontological service learning, health issues in later life, tobacco cessation in later life, minority aging, and health promotion in later life. She is author of *Respite Care: Programs, Problems and Solutions,* coauthor of *Long Term Care: Management, Scope and Practical Issues,* and 25 articles and chapters in professional journals and textbooks. Dr. Tepper is a Fellow of the Gerontological Society of America, and was a Delegate from New York to the last White House Conference on Aging.

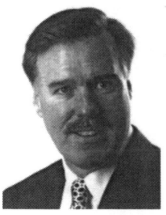

**Thomas M. Cassidy, MA,** is a Research Fellow at the American Institute for Economic Research in Great Barrington, Massachusetts, where he conducts economic research on a wide range of subjects, especially those related to the older population. Recent projects have included the Medicare Prescription Drug Act, and issues associated with elder fraud and abuse. Prior experience include a 6 year term as Senior Fellow at the Institute for Socioeconomic Studies in White Plains, New York, and almost 20 years as a senior investigator for the New York State Attorney General's Medicaid Fraud Control Unit. The third edition of his book, *Elder Care: What to Look Out For!,* was released in May, 2004. Tom has discussed elder care on PBS, NBC, CBS, CNN, FOX, and on many other television and radio programs across the country, as well as in nationally syndicated columns.

# Multidisciplinary Perspectives on Aging

**Lynn M. Tepper,** MA, MS, EdM, EdD
**Thomas M. Cassidy,** MA

Editors

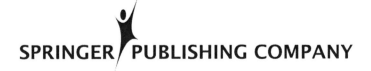

SPRINGER PUBLISHING COMPANY

Springer Publishing Company, Inc.
11 West 42nd Street, 15th Floor
New York, NY 10036-8002

*Acquisitions Editor: Ursula Springer*
*Production Editor: Janice Stangel*
*Cover design by Joanne Honigman*

05 06 07 08 / 5 4 3 2

Multidisciplinary perspectives on aging / [edited by] Lynn M. Tepper and Thomas M. Cassidy.
    p. ; cm.
    Includes bibliographical references.
    ISBN 0-8261-2575-1
    1. Older people—Care. 2. Geriatrics. 3. Gerontology.
  4. Older people—Nursing home care.
    [DNLM: 1. Health Services for the Aged—United States.
  2. Aging—United States. 3. Home for the Aged—United
States. 4. Nursing Homes—United States. 5. Social Support—
Aged—United States. WT 31 M961 2004] 1. Tepper, Lynn M.
  II. Cassidy, Thomas M.
RA564.8.M84 2004
618.97—dc22                       2004020099

Printed in the United States of America

*This book is dedicated to Jenny Tepper, Lynn Tepper's mother-in-law, who at the age of 90, embodies the essence, character, and strength of a successful, productive, and flourishing later life.*

# Contents

**PART III**
**Financial, Ethical, and Legal Issues in Elder Care**

# Contributors

**Eileen Chichin, PhD, RN,** is Co-Director of the Greenberg Center on ethics at the Jewish Home and Hospital in New York City, New York, and serves as a member of the Home's palliative care consult service. Dr. Chichin's research and educational and clinical efforts have been in the area of end-of-life ethics and palliative care, with an emphasis on the role of both professional and paraprofessional staff in these areas.

**Catherine DeLorey, RN, MPH, PhD,** is Director of the Women's Health Institute, a women's health education and communication firm in Boston, MA. She is also the National Coordinator of the Women's Universal Health Initiative, and has more than 20 years' experience as a nurse in home health care both in the US and internationally.

**Lorraine G. Hiatt, PhD,** is Director of Planning, Research, and Design for Aging in New York City, a nationally known design and planning company specializing in environments for older people. She has exhibited her designs at national conventions, the American Association of Homes and Services for the Aging, the American Institute of Architects, Design for Aging, and the Sage Nursing Homes competitions.

**Brenda M. Horrell, DDS, MS,** is Assistant Professor at Columbia University, School of Dental and Oral Surgery in New York City. She teaches oral radiology and is an integral part of the Geriatric Dentistry Program. She has presented her oral health research both nationally and internationally.

**Thomas Campbell Jackson, MPH, CEBS,** is a New York City-based health care consultant, and Director of the Galen Institute, an organization promoting public health and science literacy. He was Senior Fellow at the Institute for SocioEconomic Studies, and served as Director of New York's Health Benefits Program.

**Marshall B. Kapp, JD, MPH,** is an attorney and Professor in the Departments of Community Health and Psychiatry at the Wright State University School of Medicine, Dayton, OH. He is also a faculty member at the University of Dayton School of Law, and a Fellow of the Gerontological Society of America.

**Gary J. Kennedy, MD,** is Professor of Psychiatry and Behavioral Medicine at the Albert Einstein College of Medicine, and Montifiore Medical Center, New York City, where he is Director of Geriatric Psychiatry. He is a Fellow of the Brookdale Center on Aging of Hunter College, and has received numerous awards from gerontological professional organizations.

**Colin Kopes-Kerr, MD, JD, MPH,** is Vice Chairman and Residency Program Director at SUNY Stony Brook Department of Family Medicine. His major areas of interest and research are evidence-based medicine, quality assurance in primary care, computers in primary care, and quality assurance for diabetes.

**Patricia A. Miller, EdD, OTR, FAOTA,** is Associate Professor at Columbia University, College of Physicians and Surgeons, Program in Occupational Therapy. She is a consultant to local, state, and national organizations in interdisciplinary teamwork, fall prevention, program development for community agencies serving the elderly, and assessment and treatment of depression.

**Sally S. Robinson, LMSW, PhD,** is a bereavement support therapist at the Hospice of Kershaw County Medical Center in Camden, SC. She was the Founder and Executive Director of the City of Yonkers Office for the Aging, developing and administering a comprehensive array of community services to older adults and their families.

**Richard H. Rubin, MD,** is Professor of Medicine at the University of New Mexico, Health Sciences Center, and Fellow in the American College of Physicians. He is Co-Editor of *Medicine: A Primary Care Approach,* a textbook of ambulatory medicine for medical students.

**William T. Smith, MSW, PhD,** is the President and CEO of Aging in America in the Bronx, New York, and Chairman of the American Association of Homes and Services for the Aging. He has practiced social work for 28 years, and administered and developed long-term care organizations including nursing homes, home- and community-based programs, and housing services for seniors.

# Preface

The dawn of the twenty-first century is an exciting time to experience the enormous changes that have had a positive effect on all aspects of our lives. The dramatic advancements in science and technology have added both quality and quantity to our lives. However, the demographic shift that has taken place has called forth a need to explore its implications. The aging of the massive numbers of people who are often referred to as the "Baby-Boomer Population," those born between 1946 and 1964, will have huge implications for society as well as for individuals. Combined with the phenomenon of substantially increased life expectancy, we have outcomes producing extensive concerns for professionals in a variety of settings.

It was these extensive, yet differing effects of the huge "elder-boom" that provided the first inspiration for a book of this kind. The authors wanted to put together a comprehensive textbook that focused on a multidisciplinary approach for providing services to older people, a book that can be used by students in diverse programs who want to understand, from a variety of perspectives, what needs to be done.

The inspiration for this book has also come from the array of experiences of its authors. The editors, Lynn Tepper and Thomas Cassidy, represent two very different disciplines and two very different occupational backgrounds. Lynn is a gerontologist and professor with many years of teaching, research, and clinical experience with older people, and Tom, a former Senior Special Investigator with the New York State Attorney General's Office, specializes in elder abuse and institutional care, and is a researcher in economic issues and policies facing the elderly.

When Lynn Tepper and Tom Cassidy met, Tom was writing his first book, *Elder Care: What to Look For, What to Look Out For* (1997). Lynn had been recommended by several of Tom's colleagues as a recognized leader in gerontology, and someone who could provide some insight into the complexity of elder care issues. It did not take long for the perspectives of each to be shared and appreciated by the other, and to recognize their common goal: quality of life for older people.

This book represents the efforts of both to write about their own concerns, experiences, and issues facing older people, but equally important, to draw upon the background and experiences of other recognized leaders in fields that impact greatly upon the needs of our older population. They hope it will be valuable to students in a variety of professional capacities—social services, health care, public health, mental health, health services administration, planning and design—and all future providers and advocates for the needs of our older population.

# Acknowledgments

T he editors most gratefully acknowledge their fellow contributors, whose vast knowledge about each of their disciplines has come together to produce this book. They are a very special group of professionals who, although different in their approaches to aging issues, are united in their appreciation of the need for collaboration and teamwork in helping older people live to their potential best.

Lynn Tepper is especially grateful to Dr. Ruth Bennett, her mentor and former professor at Columbia University, who first opened her eyes to the need for those caring for older people to listen to each other and appreciate what each has to contribute to elders' total well-being. Dr. Bennett continues to demonstrate that careful planning combined with intellectual curiosity can perpetuate a meaningful and productive life after retirement.

Tom Cassidy is appreciative to Fred S. Sganga, Executive Director at the Long Island State Veterans Home at Stony Brook University, and Julian Rich, President/CEO of Penacook Place for sharing their knowledge and enthusiasm.

Both authors are appreciative to Dr. William Tepper, who provided valuable content feedback about each chapter from the perspective of someone outside the field of gerontology. The meticulous editorial and organizational skills of Lauren Dockett of Springer Publishing Company enabled this book to go to press in a well-structured and comprehensible format. Dr. Ursula Springer is to be thanked for enthusiasm and support of this book from its conception.

# Part I

## Changing Relationships, Changing Care Needs

# Aging in America:
# Challenges and Opportunities

## *Lynn M. Tepper*

Older people in the twenty-first century have often been referred to as the "new-old," in that they are very different from previous generations of older people in many ways. In addition to being the fastest growing age group, they are also an important segment of our population, as they bring with them many challenges and opportunities. This text contains some of the most important of these issues that older people face: housing, finance, legal concerns, environmental needs, physical health, mental health, changing family relationships, abuse and neglect, ethical considerations, and end-of-life care needs.

Who are these elderly that everyone is so concerned about? How are they faring overall? How are they in respect to health and well-being? This introductory chapter will present a brief overview of some of the key indicators about older Americans: a representation of current, twenty-first-century data on the status of this group.

At the beginning of this new century, we find that older Americans are living longer and enjoying greater prosperity than any previous generation. They are also the best educated of any previous cohort, and are the healthiest group of older people on record since data have been collected on these issues. However, with new opportunities that come with advanced scientific progress also come challenges. Despite these advances, persistent inequalities between the sexes, income classes, and racial and ethnic groups continue to exist (Federal Forum on Aging Related Statistics, 2000). In only a few years, the oldest of the "baby-boom" population (the result of a massive increase in birthrate between 1946 and 1964) will turn 65. For more than 50 years, demographers have known that we would be experiencing a large "bulge" in the population created by the deferral of childbearing during World

War II, and the relative prosperity that followed. This population cohort of 76 million has the full attention of the health care profession, work force planners, financial advisors, community leaders, policy makers, researchers, human ecologists, program planners, and public benefit agencies. Challenges have already been experienced in public policy and the mature marketplace (U.S. Department of Health and Human Services, 2003a). These challenges intensify the need for us all to better understand the health and economic needs of older Americans and their implications.

## DEMOGRAPHICS AND LIFE EXPECTANCY

Over the last one hundred years, advances in sanitation, nutrition, and medical knowledge have made possible great changes in life expectancy in the United States and throughout many part of the world. It is important to distinguish between two related concepts: life span and life expectancy. The maximum human *life span*, currently 124, is the potential number of years that could be attained if an individual were able to avoid or be successfully treated for all illnesses and accidents. Actually, as recent research has created the possibility of altering the genetic code, the possibility of extending currently accepted limits of human life beyond 124 years is raised (National Institutes of Health, 2002). This differs from *life expectancy*, which is the age by which a population born at a certain time is expected to die. A child born in 1900 had a life expectancy of 47.3 years, whereas a child born in 2003 can expect to live until the age of 77.2–79.8 for women and 74.4 for men (U.S. Department of Health and Human Services, 2003b). However, life expectancy rises with age, which means that under current mortality conditions, people who survive to 65 can expect to live an average of nearly 20 more years; to 75, another 12 years; and to 85, another 7 years (National Vital Statistics Report, 2002). Life expectancy varies by race, but the difference decreases with age. For example, life expectancy is now six years higher for white persons than for black persons. However, black persons outlive whites among those who survive to age 85. When we consider the *proportion* of the total population, the data is even more overwhelming: In 1900 the percentage of those over 65 in the total population was a mere 3%; in 2001 it rose to 12.4%. In *numbers* this represents a growth from 3 million in 1900 to a more than a ten-fold increase to 35 million in 2001.

## FUTURE GROWTH

The older population is expected to increase significantly during the next 30 years. This growth slowed somewhat during the 1990s because of the relatively small number of babies born during the Great Depression of the 1930s. But the older population will burgeon between the years 2010 and 2030 when the baby boom generation reaches 65. The population will double from a present 35 million to 70 million. This number will rise again significantly in 2050 to a projected 82 million (Fig. 1.1).

The present 12.4 percent of our population will jump to 20 percent by 2030. Even more startling is the rapidly growing number of people over the age of 85, by far the fastest growing segment of the older population. This group will grow from 1.6 percent in 2001 to 2.5 percent in 2030 and 4.3 percent in 2050. In numbers, this means a growth from 4.2 million in 2001 to 8.9 million in 2030 (U.S. Administration on Aging, 2002; www.census.gov/population/projections, 2002). The size of this group is especially important for the future of our health care system, as these individuals tend to be in poorer health and require more services than do the younger old (Federal Forum on Aging Related Statistics, 2000).

Public interest in life extension is currently on the rise. Products and services to reverse or delay onset of normal aging are on the increase, as can be observed in the print media, television, and Internet sites, which focus on anti-aging and life-extension food supplements, plastic surgery, and cosmetic products. Marketing to this growing population has become part of corporate objectives, and even academia, with such courses as Elder Care Marketing and Retirement Planning as part of business school curricula.

## MARITAL STATUS

Marriages of forty or more years have become much more common among the current cohort of older people. Older couples in long-term marriages are far less likely to divorce than younger ones. Overall, marital satisfaction has been measured highest in early years and later years of marriage (Berry & Williams, 1987). Older couples may in fact have different criteria for marital satisfaction than do younger couples (Tepper, 1994).

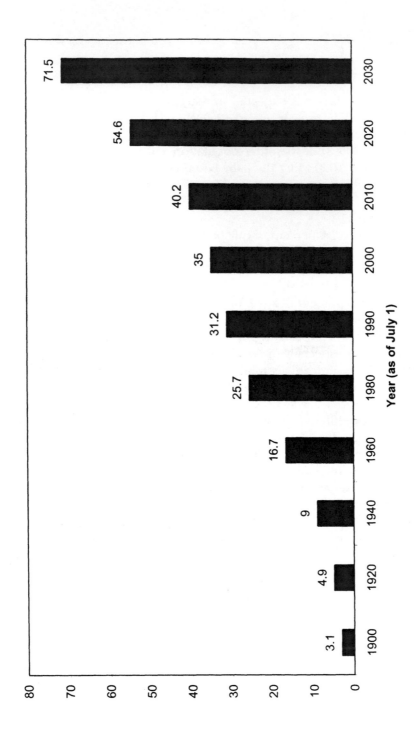

**FIGURE 1.1  Number of persons 65+, 1990–2030 (in millions).**

*Source:* U.S. Bureau of the Census, Current Population Reports, Census Internet Release, January, 2004

A substantial percentage of the older population is widowed. Not surprisingly, women are much more likely than men to experience the death of a spouse. In 1998, about 77 percent of women age 85 or older were widowed, compared with 42 percent of men. Widows outnumber widowers nearly six to one (U.S. Bureau of the Census, 2000a), but seem to adjust better than men to the death of a spouse. As it is, they represent 58 percent of the population 65 and over and 70 percent of those 85 and over (U.S. Administration on Aging, 2002), so are more likely to survive their spouse based on differences in life expectancy, the tendency for women to marry men who are older, and higher remarriage rates for older widowed men than widowed women. In 2001, older men were much more likely to be married—73 percent of men, 41 percent of women. Almost half of all older women in 2001 (46%) were widows (U.S. Administration on Aging, 2002). Marital status often affects an individual's emotional and economic well-being by influencing living arrangements and availability of caregivers among older people with an illness or disability. According to census reports, divorce rates amount to only 7 percent of the older population, and only a small percentage never marry: 4 percent of women and 4 percent of men (U.S. Census, March, 2002; see Fig. 1.2).

## LIVING ARRANGEMENTS

Although much of the research on living environments of the elderly has focused on nursing homes, public housing, or retirement communities, the proportion of older people in these living conditions is actually very small. The vast majority—95 percent—of persons 65 and over are living in the community, rather than in institutions. Of the 35 million older people in the population, the U.S. Census recorded 22 million living in family homes, 10 million of them alone (U.S. Bureau of the Census, 2000a). Over half (55%) of the older community residents lived with their spouse in 2000. The proportion living with spouses decreased with age, especially for women. Only 28.8 percent of women 75 and over lived with a spouse (U.S. Administration on Aging, 2002). Among other older people, 7 percent lived with other relatives, 3 percent lived with non-relatives, and 30 percent lived alone.

Where and with whom one lives are important considerations because they are closely linked to income, health status, and the availability of caregivers. Older persons who live alone are more likely to be in poverty than those who reside with their spouses (Dalaker, 1999). When we consider gender, older women are more likely to live alone. In 2000,

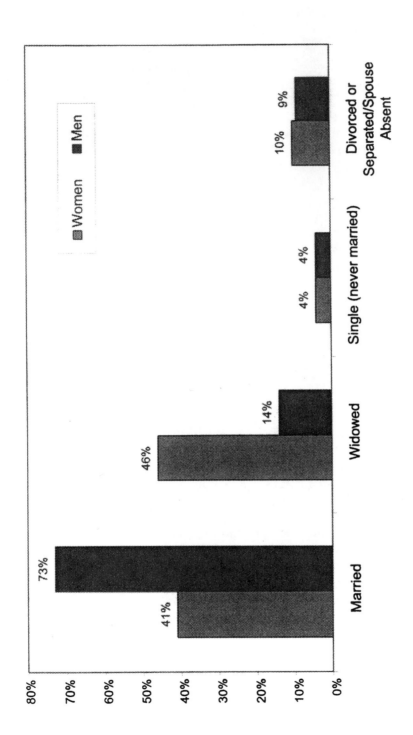

**FIGURE 1.2  Marital status of persons 65+ in 2001.**

*Source:* U.S. Bureau of the Census, 2002a

8

40 percent of elders living alone were women and only 17 percent were men. When we consider race, we see some differences as well. About 40 percent of both older white and older black women lived alone, compared with only 27 percent of older Hispanic women, and 21 percent of older Asian and Pacific Islander women. Whereas 15 percent of older white women lived with other relatives, approximately one third of older black, Asian and Pacific Islander, and Hispanic women lived with other relatives. Poverty rates are higher for older women who live alone than they are for older women who live with a spouse. We now see about 20 percent of white older women who live alone in poverty, and approximately 50 percent of older black and Hispanic women living in poverty (U.S. Bureau of the Census, 2000b).

Nursing homes may be the only alternative for some older adults with serious, chronic health problems. A small percentage, 5% (1.56 million), of the older population lived in institutions in 2001, but the percentage increases dramatically with age, ranging from 1.1 percent for persons 65–74 years to 4.7 percent for persons 75–84 years, and 1.8 percent for the 85 and over group (U.S. Administration on Aging, 2003). However, significant advances in the delivery of home health care services have increased the number of frail elders in poor health receiving care in their homes, rather than in institutions.

## ETHNIC AND RACIAL COMPOSITION

As the older population increases, it will also grow more diverse, reflecting the demographic changes in the U.S. population as a whole over the past century. Even within ethnic groups there is diversity. These differences are related largely to length of time in the U.S. and socioeconomic status, both of which affect assimilation and the relative degree of cultural identity. Many of the formerly disadvantaged minority population are now gaining access to a higher standard of living that accompanies expanded opportunities and access to better health care (Gutheil & Tepper, 1994). In 2002, 83.6 percent of the population 65 and over were white, 8 percent were black, 2.5 percent were non-Hispanic Asian and Pacific Islander, and less than 1 percent was American Indian and Native Alaskan. Of this population, .8 percent identified themselves as being of two or more races. The white population is expected to decline from 83.6 percent to 64 percent by 2050. Older Hispanics are among the fastest growing population, increasing from a present 6 percent to an expected 16 percent by 2050. In numbers, they represent the largest increase: from 2 million to over 13 million by 2050. It is projected that Hispanic elderly will outnumber black elderly by 2028. Asian and Pacific Islanders will increase from 2 percent to 7 percent. The black population will grow from 8 percent to 12 percent, and we will experience only negligible growth among other smaller minority populations (U.S. Bureau of the Census, 2003).

An understanding and respect for the culture of each group—their behaviors, attitudes, and values—is an important part of providing all types of services. Within the next 50 years, programs and services for the older population will require greater flexibility to meet the demands of a diverse and changing population.

## EDUCATION

The current generation of older Americans is far better educated than previous generations, and this trend will continue. Educational attainment often influences socioeconomic status, and therefore plays an important role in well-being at older ages. More education is usually associated with higher incomes, higher standards of living, and above-average health status among older adults. For example, in 1950 only 17.7 percent of older people had finished high school. In 2002, the number rose to 69.9 percent. Those with a bachelors degree or higher increased from 3.6 percent in 1950 to 16.7 percent in 2002 (11 percent of older women and 20 percent of older men) (www.agingstats.gov, 2003). Despite these large overall increases in educational level among older adults, when we consider race and ethnicity, many differences can be noted. In 2002, 74.3 percent of the white population 65 and over had finished high school, compared to 68 percent of the Asian and Pacific Islanders, 50 percent of blacks, and 35.3 percent of Hispanics. College completion rates are 17.9 percent of the older white population, 24.2 percent of Asian and Pacific Islanders, 10.3 percent of blacks, and 5.5 percent of Hispanics 65 and over (www.agingstats.gov, 2003).

The future elderly will be the best educated in history. Over half of this age group has graduated from high school, and almost a quarter have a college education. Increased education has vast socioeconomic implications and expanded opportunities for these future elders. For example, senior housing, retirement communities, and assisted living facilities will have to include high speed Internet access to meet the market need.

## POVERTY

Officially, the measure of poverty is based on a family's annual income. Presently, the official poverty level is $8,980 per year income per one person household (www.agingstats.gov, 2003). People of all ages living in poverty are at risk of having inadequate resources for food, housing, health care, and other needs. Before the enactment of the Older Americans Act in 1965, the first Federal legislation that established entitlements, benefits, and programs specifically for the population over 65, the poverty rate for this population was 28.5 percent, almost three times that of the population under 65. By 2002, the percentage of older people living in poverty declined to 10.1 percent, roughly the same as those of working age. Among older people, the poverty rate is higher at older ages. It is presently 9.2 percent for persons 65 to 74, 10.4 percent for persons aged 75 to 84, and 13.0 percent for those 85 and older. Among the older population, poverty rates are higher among women (12.4 percent) than among men (7 percent); among the non-married (16.9 percent) compared with the married (4.7 percent); and among minorities (21.9 percent) compared with white persons (8.1 percent) (Federal Interagency Forum on Aging Related Statistics, 2003). Presently divorced black women ages 65 to 74 had a poverty rate of 47 percent, one of the highest rates for any subgroup of older people (U.S. Bureau of the Census, 2002b).

## THE ECONOMICS OF AGING

The age composition of a society in part determines the allocation of its resources. As has been discussed, the progressively older population over the next 50 years will require more financial resources to meet its needs. What is profoundly changing in this country is the dependency ratio, the ratio of workers to those retirees dependent on them. By 2020, there will be more adults over 65 than under 18. How to distribute the economic resources needed to support young and old, especially when health costs are rapidly increasing, will pose real challenges for policy makers.

### Income

The median income of older persons in 2002 was $14,152: $19,688 for males and $11,313 for females (Federal Registry, 2003). However, real median income after adjustment for inflation fell by −2.6 percent since 2000 (U.S. Administration on Aging, 2002). Poverty rates have declined over the past 30 years, as have the numbers of low-income elderly from 34.6 percent to 28.1 percent. Medium- and high-income elders have increased from 50.8 percent to almost 61.9 percent (www.agingstats.gov, 2003). High-income elders have especially increased over these years, making the current cohort of older people in the best shape financially of all previous generations of elders (Fig. 1.3).

### Net Worth

Great disparities exist which is reflected most clearly when we consider the values of real estate, stocks, bonds, and other assets, minus outstanding debts, of this population. Net worth is an important indicator of economic security and well-being. Greater net worth allows a family to maintain its standard of living when income falls because of retirement, job loss, health problems, or family changes such as divorce or widowhood. In the past 20 years the median net worth among households headed by persons age 65 or older increased by almost 87.7 percent, whereas the median net worth for households headed by persons ages 45 to 64 declined by 20.5 percent. Most striking is the disparity in net worth between black and white households headed by persons 65 and over. Presently, median net worth among older black households is $40,100, compared with $207,700 among older white households (Federal Interagency Forum on Aging Related Statistics, 2003).

When we consider the income of households headed by persons 65 and over in 2002, the median income was $33,802. About one in nine households had income less than $15,000, and 45 percent had incomes of $35,000 or more (U.S. Administration on Aging, 2003; Fig. 1.4).

Educational attainment is the most important indicator found to affect net worth. With this enormous growth of the older population comes the increased need to reflect upon our public policies in place for this group. Expanded support for its neediest elders and expanded marketing opportunities for its wealthiest are both challenges and opportunities for our society.

### MORTALITY

Death rates for the total population have declined over the past century. However, for some diseases, death rates among older people have re-

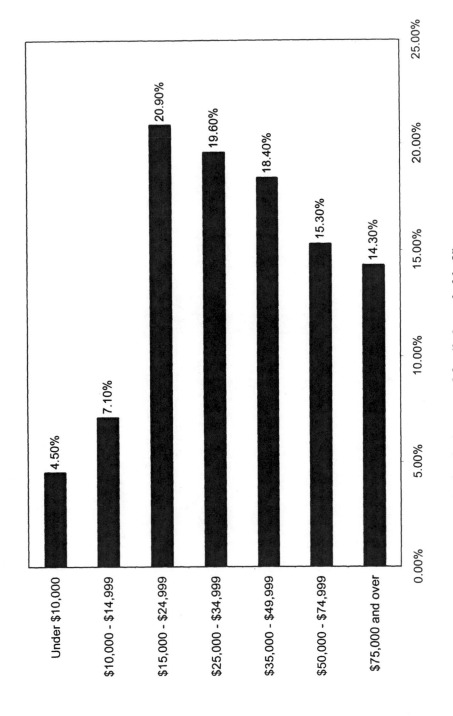

**FIGURE 1.3  Percent distribution by income of family households 65+.**

*Source:* U.S. Administration on Aging, A Profile of Older Americans: 2003

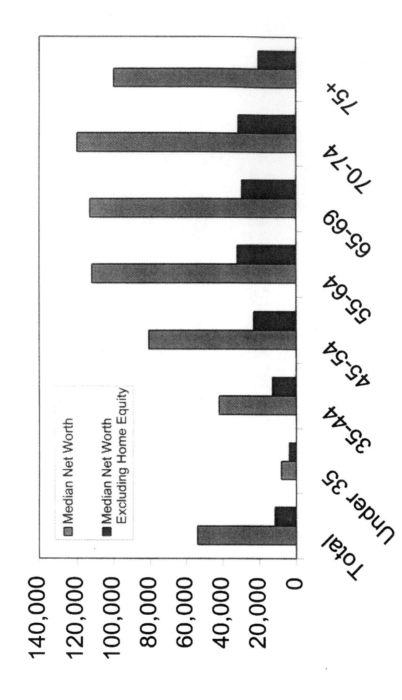

**FIGURE 1.4  Median net worth of households with householder 65+.**

*Source:* Current Population Reports, Net Worth and Ownership of Households: 2000, pp 70–88, May 2003.

cently increased. For example, between 1980 and today, age-adjusted death rates for heart disease and stroke declined by approximately one-third. However, death rates for cancer, pneumonia, and influenza increased slightly over the same period. Death rates for diabetes increased by 32 percent and for chronic obstructive pulmonary diseases by 57 percent. Today, the leading cause of death among older persons is heart disease, followed by cancer, stroke, pulmonary disease, pneumonia and influenza, and diabetes (National Center for Health Statistics, 2003). Alzheimer's disease was the sixth leading cause of death among white women 85 and over; however it was less common among black women the same age group or men of either race.

A number of studies have found a positive relationship among social networks, social support, health indicators, and lower mortality rates among the elderly. Higher mortality rate is affected by several factors, for both men and women, including having fewer children and belonging to fewer organizations (Tucker, Schwartz, Clark, & Friedman, 1999).

## HEALTH STATUS

Among the older population, chronic diseases that bring with them long-term illness and are rarely cured profoundly influence quality of life. These conditions can become a significant health and financial burden not only to those persons who have them, but also to their families and the nation's health care system. Chronic conditions such as arthritis, diabetes, and heart disease negatively affect quality of life, contributing to declines in functioning and frequently the inability to remain in the community (Centers for Disease Control and Prevention, 2000).

Most older persons have at least one chronic condition and many have multiple conditions. The most frequently occurring conditions per 100 elderly in 1996 were arthritis (49), hypertension (36), hearing impairment (30), heart disease (27), cataracts (17), orthopedic impairments (18), sinusitis (12), and diabetes (10). Increased longevity for many older people has brought with it increasing years of chronic health conditions and frailty. Treating this group remains a challenge for medical professionals, with the goal of optimal functioning often replacing cure.

## MENTAL HEALTH

Mental health implies the absence of psychological disorders and the positive outcomes of coping and adaptation (Hoyer & Roodin, 2003).

However, because advanced age is usually coupled with increased physical illness, physical and mental health are more interwoven in later life. This problem is even more intensified by the fact that older people with mental health problems are less likely to receive help than younger people (Gatz, 2000).

Depressive symptoms are an important indicator of general well-being and mental health. Among all ages, higher levels of depressive symptoms are associated with higher rates of physical illness, greater functional disability, and higher health care resource utilization. Women between 65 and 84 are more likely than men to have severe depressive symptoms (18 percent compared to 10 percent). Among persons 85 and older, men and women have a similar prevalence of severe depressive symptoms, accounting for as high as 23 percent (Wells et al., 1989). The rate of depression increases with age in all studies.

Closely related to depression is higher risk for alcoholism and suicide, both of which are known to increase with age. The sharp increase in suicide is most notable among white males 85 and over, who have six times the suicide rate of the general public (Lebowitz et al., 1997).

Memory skills are important to general cognitive functioning, and declining scores on tests of memory are indicators of general cognitive loss for older adults. Low cognitive functioning is a major risk factor for entering a nursing home (Wygaard & Albreksten, 1992). However, the proportion of older people with moderate or severe memory impairment ranged from about 4 percent among the 65–74-year-olds, to about 36 percent among persons age 85 or older (Federal Interagency Forum on Aging Related Statistics, 2003). These data support the need to dispel the myth that dementia is part of normal aging, as a majority of elders have cognitive function that does not limit their quality of life.

## DISABILITY

Functioning in later years may be diminished if illness, chronic disease, or injury limits physical and/or mental abilities. Changes in disability rates have important implications for work and retirement policies, health and long-term care needs, and the social well-being of the older population. By monitoring and understanding these trends, policymakers are better able to make informed decisions. Different indicators can be used to monitor disability including limitations in Activities of Daily Living (ADLs) and Instrumental Activities of Daily Living (IADLs), and measure of physical, cognitive, and social functioning. Aspects of physical functioning such as the ability to climb stairs, walk a quarter mile, or reach up over one's head are more closely linked to physiological capabilities than are ADLs or IADLs, which may be influenced by social and cultural role expectations and by changes in technology. Trend data on disability and age suggest that on the average, persons of a given age are healthier and have fewer disabling conditions than others of the same age did ten years before. However, because disabilities increase with age, and our population is living longer, the number of individuals with activity, work, or functional limitations is increasing (U.S. Administration on Aging, 2002). In the past twenty years we have seen a decline in disability from 24 percent to 21 percent. However, despite the decline rates, the number of older people with chronic disabilities increased by about 600,000 from 6.4 million to over 7 million. This reflects the fast growth rate of this population, enough to outweigh the decline in disability rates (Fig. 1.5).

From 1975 to 1995, both older men and older women reported improvements in physical functioning in the ability to walk a quarter mile, climb stairs, reach up over their heads, and stoop, crouch, or kneel. In 1995, older black persons (33 percent) were more likely than older whites (25 percent) to be unable to perform at least one of nine physical activities (National Center for Health Statistics, 1995).

## HEALTH PROMOTION AND DISEASE PREVENTION

The twentieth century brought with it research resulting in the realization that promoting health and preventing disease are within the capabilities of people of all ages. There is increasing evidence that links lifestyle choices to longevity and good health in the later years (U.S. Department of Health and Human Services, 2003a). The relationship among social, emotional, and physical health were also a product of twentieth-century research and practice.

Men and women benefit from social activities at all ages. Those who continue to interact with others tend to be healthier, both physically and mentally, than those who become socially isolated. Interactions with friends and family members can provide emotional and practical support that enables older people to remain in the community and reduce the likelihood they will need formal health care services.

Physical activity is also beneficial for the health and well-being of all ages. It can reduce the risk of certain chronic diseases, may relieve symptoms of depression, helps to maintain independent living, and enhances overall quality of life (U.S. Department of Health and Human

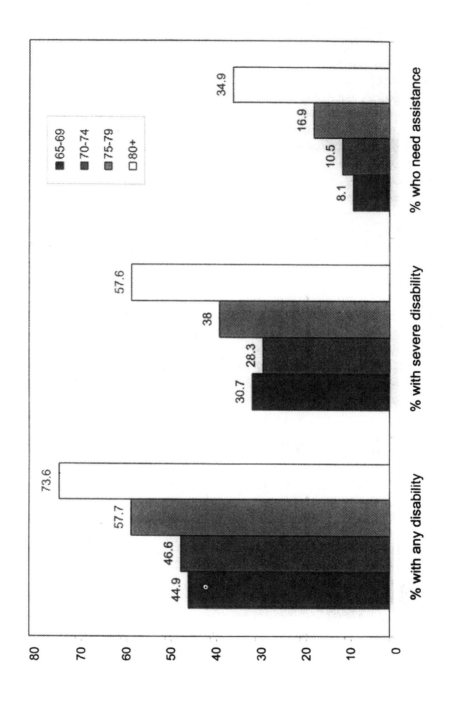

**FIGURE 1.5  Percent of older people with disability by age.**

*Source:* U.S. Administration on Aging, A Profile of Older Americans: 2003

Services, 1996). Research has shown that even among frail and very old adults 85 and over, mobility and functioning can be improved through physical activity (Butler, Davis, Lewis, Nelson, & Strauss, 1998).

Vaccinations against influenza and pneumonia are recommended for older people, who are at increased risk for complications from these diseases compared with younger individuals. The costs of these vaccinations are covered under both Medicaid and Medicare. Health services and screenings can help prevent disease or detect it at an early, possibly treatable stage. Mammography, colonoscopy, and prostate examination are examples of preventive screenings, also covered under the above federal insurance policies.

Dietary quality plays a major role in preventing or delaying the onset of chronic diseases. Various health indexes are used to rate healthy eating behaviors. A government survey indicated that diets were rated "good" for a higher percentage of the 65 and over age group (13 percent) than for middle-aged persons aged 45 to 64 (9 percent). Even so, a majority of older persons (67 percent) report diets that need improvement (Tippet & Cypel, 1998).

## HEALTH CARE: FINANCING

Health can be a major expense for people as they age, especially for those with limited income who have a chronic condition or disability. Expenditures on health care include the cost of medical professionals' services, hospitalizations, home health care, nursing home care, medications, and any other goods and services used in the treatment or prevention of disease. In 2002, the average annual expenditure on health care for older people was $3,493 in out-of-pocket expenditures: $5,864 among people 65 to 69, compared with $9, 414 among 75–79-year-olds, and $16,465 among persons age 85 and over. This represents an increase of more than half since 1990. In contrast, the total population spent considerably less, averaging $2,182 in out-of-pocket costs. Older people spent 12.6 percent of their total expenditures on health, more than twice the proportion spent by all consumers (5.5 percent) (U.S. Administration on Aging, 2002). Choosing between food and medication can be a result of this phenomenon, when affording both is not possible.

Older people living in institutions incurred an average of $40,000 in annual health care expenditures, compared with an average of $6,400 among those living in the community. The costs of health care continue to increase annually and are concentrated among a relatively small group of individuals. About 1% of Medicare beneficiaries age 65 or older incur 13 percent of the health care expenditures in that group. The top 5 percent of enrollees with the highest expenditures incurred 37 percent of all health care expenditures. People 85 and over continue to spend the most on health care in all categories: nursing home, home health, hospitalization, medical outpatient, and prescriptions. Of all Medicare beneficiaries living in the community, about 70 percent have prescription coverage through HMO, Medicaid, or private Medicare supplements. Those who did not have this coverage had 83 percent higher out-of-pocket expenses than those with drug coverage (Poisal & Chulis, 2000). Improved coverage for prescription drugs continues to be an important health care policy priority, with recent changes providing Medicare recipients with 10–15% off drug prices, or as much as $600 yearly (American Association of Retired Persons, 2003).

## HEALTH CARE: ACCESS

Access to health care is determined by a variety of factors related to the cost, quality, and availability of services. Over 96 percent of older people are covered by Medicare, which provides affordable coverage for most acute health care services. However, health care users also require a reliable source of care that is provided without major inconvenience. The percentage of older people reporting difficulty in obtaining health care was down from 3 percent in 1992 to 2 percent in 1998. Those who reported delaying the use of health care because of cost declined from 10 percent to 6 percent. Access to health care varies by race. The group reporting highest delays based on cost were black elders (10 percent), followed by Hispanics (7 percent), and whites (5 percent) (Centers for Medicare and Medicaid Services, 2003). Most older people have access to health care through Medicare, providing access to a variety of services, including inpatient hospital care, physician care, outpatient care, home health care, and limited care at a nursing home. However the types of health services that older people receive under Medicare have changed over the past decade, and there are many limitations on some of these payments.

## HEALTH CARE: UTILIZATION

Physician visits have increased more than 30 percent in the last 10 years, as have home health care services, with an enormous four-fold increase. Only a moderate increase has been noted in hospital admissions over these years; however admissions to nursing homes have risen from 23 admissions per 1,000 people to 70 per 1,000 people. As can be expected, the use of home health care and nursing home care increases markedly with age. In 1998, home health care agencies made 2,350 home health visits per 1,000 persons ages 65 to 74, compared with 12,709 among persons age 85 or over. Similarly, nursing home admissions per 1,000 people were 27 for the 65–74 age group and 200 for persons 85 and over (Health Care Financing Administration, 1999).

We are seeing higher health care utilization patterns than ever before. Older people had about four times the number of days of hospitalization than did those under 65 in 2000. The average length of a hospital stay was 6.4 days for older people, compared to 4.6 days for people of all ages. The average length of stay for older people has decreased 6 days since 1964. Older people averaged many more contacts with doctors in 2000 than did persons of all ages: 7 contacts vs. 3.7 contacts (U.S. Administration on Aging, 2002).

## CONCLUSION

The twenty-first century has brought with it enormous scientific and technological advancement which has improved the quality of life for many people who directly benefit from these advances. The opportunities for older adults have increased dramatically, bringing with them challenges to all of us who are in a position to improve the well-being of this population. It is in this context that all professionals who directly or indirectly have an effect on older people must rethink the goals that their profession has set forth. The multiple and complex needs of our older population also brings with it a need to understand, appreciate, and consider the roles and perspectives of other disciplines, as they pertain to improving the well-being of elders, and ourselves as we age.

## REFERENCES

American Association of Retired Persons. (2003). What does the new Medicare drug benefit mean for you? www.aarp.org. Washington, DC.

Berry, R. E., & Williams, F. L. (1987). Assessing the relationship between quality of life and marital and income satisfaction. *Journal of Marriage and the Family*, *49*, 107–116.

Butler, R. N., Davis, R., Lewis, C. B., Nelson, M. E., & Strauss, E. (1998). Physical fitness: Benefits of exercise for the older patient. *Geriatrics*, *53*(10), 46–62.

Centers for Disease Control and Prevention. (2000). *Unrealized prevention opportunities: Reducing the health and economic burden of chronic disease.* Atlanta: Author.

Centers for Medicare and Medicaid Services. (2003). *National Health Statistics Report.* www.cms.hhs.gov/statistics

Dalaker, J. (1999). Poverty in the United States: 1998. U.S. Census Bureau, *Current population reports.* P60–207. Washington, DC: U.S. Government Printing Office.

Federal Forum on Aging Related Statistics. (2000). *Older Americans 2000: Key indicators of well-being.* Hyattsville, MD: National Center for Heath Statistics.

Federal Forum on Aging Related Statistics. (2002). *Current population survey supplement,* www.agingstats.gov/tables

Federal Interagency Forum on Aging-Related Statistics. (2003). *Older Americans 2003: Key indicators of well-being.* Hyattsville, MD: National Center for Health Services.

Federal Registry. (February 7, 2003). Vol. 68, No. 26, 6456-6458.

Gatz, M. (2000). Contemporary geropsychology. *The Gerontologist, 40*(5), 627–629.

Gutheil, I. A., & Tepper, L. M. (1994). The aging family: Ethnic and cultural considerations. In E. P. Congress (Ed.), *Multicultural perspectives in working with families* (pp. 89–105). New York: Springer.

Health Care Financing Administration. (1999). *A profile of Medicare home health: Chart book.* Report # 1999-771-472. Washington, DC: U.S. Government Printing Office.

Hoyer, W. J., & Roodin, P. A. (2003). *Adult development and aging.* New York: McGraw Hill.

Lebowitz, B. D., Pearson, J. L., Schneider, L. S., Reynolds, C. F., Alexopoulos, P. S., Bruce, M. L., Conwell, Y., Katz, I. R., Meyers, B. S., Morrison, M. F., Mossey, J., Niederehe, G., & Parmelee, P. (1997). Diagnosis and treatment of depression in late life: Consensus statement update. *Journal of the American Medical Association, 278*(14), 1186–1190.

National Center for Health Statistics. (1995). *Supplement on aging II.* Atlanta: Centers for Disease Control and Prevention, National Center for Health Statistics.

National Center for Health Statistics. (2000). *Health, United States, 1999, with health and aging chartbook* (pp. 36–37). Hyattsville, MD: Author.

National Center for Health Statistics. (2003). Deaths: Final data, 2001. In E. Arias, R. N. Anderson, H. C. Kung, et al., *National vital statistics reports,* Vol. 52, No. 3. Hyattsville, MD.

National Institutes of Health. (2002). *Longevity.* Administration on Aging, Aging Internet Information Notes. www.nih.gov/health/agepages/lifeext.htm

National Vital Statistics Report. (2002, December). *Life expectancy by age, race, and sex, 1919 to 2001,* Vol. 51, No. 3. Hyattsville, MD.

Poisal, J. S., & Chulis, G. S. (2000). Medicare beneficiaries and drug coverage. *Health Affairs, 19*(2), 248–256.

Tepper, L. M. (1994). Family relationships in later life. In I. A. Gutheil (Ed.), *Work with older people* (pp. 42–62). New York: Fordham University Press.

Tippet, K. S., & Cypel, Y. S. (1998). *The continuing survey of food intakes by individuals and the diet and health knowledge survey.* U.S. Department of Agriculture, Agricultural Research Service, NFS Rep. No. 96-1.

Tucker, J. S., Schwartz, J. E., Clark, K. M., & Friedman, H. W. (1999). Age related changes in the associations of social network ties with mortality risk. *Psychology and Aging, 4,* 564–571.

U.S. Administration on Aging. (2002). *A profile of older Americans 2002.* Hyattsville, MD: U.S. Department of Health and Human Services.

U.S. Administration on Aging. (2003). *A profile of older Americans 2003.* Hyattsville, MD: U.S. Department of Health and Human Services.

U.S. Bureau of the Census (2002a). *Current population survey reports: Marital status and living arrangements* P20-484. Washington, DC: U.S. Government Printing Office.

U.S. Bureau of the Census. (2002b). *Poverty in the United States, 2001*, Tables 60-219.

U.S. Bureau of the Census. (2004). *Current population reports.* www.census.gov/population/projections

U.S. Department of Health and Human Services. (1996). *Physical activity and health: A report of the Surgeon General.* Atlanta: Centers for Disease Control and Prevention, National Center for Chronic Disease Prevention and Health Promotion.

U.S. Department of Health and Human Services. (2003a). *Aging Internet information notes: Baby boomers.* www.aoa.gov

U.S. Department of Health and Human Services. (2003b). Study finds life expectancy rose to 77.2 years in 2002. *Health and Human Service News*, March 14. www.hhs.gov

Wells, K. B., Stewart, A., Hayes, R. D., Burman, A., Rogers, W., Daniels, M., Berry, S., Greenfield, S., & Ware, J. (1989). The functioning and well-being of depressed patients. *Journal of the American Medical Association, 262*, 914–919.

Wygaard, H. A., & Albreksten, G. (1992). Risk factors for admission to a nursing home. A study of elderly people receiving home nursing. *Journal of Primary Health Care, 10*, 128–133.

# 2

# Family Relationships and Support Networks

## Lynn M. Tepper

Twenty-first century families are alive and well, and in reality do not fulfill the prophecy of doom imposed upon them by public opinion. Family relationships can run the gamut from violence to unconditional love, and are capable of being both the greatest source of pain and the greatest opportunity for joy (Tepper, 1994). They influence our lives from the time we are very young children to the time we reach old age. The demography of the family system varies widely. Some older people have large and extensive families, with relatives nearby, and some have very few or no family at all, managing to outlive siblings, spouses, children, and other relatives. The contemporary family is also diverse, and can include sons and daughters from previous marriages, single-parent families, and same sex or opposite sex partners, grandparents, great-grandparents, and so forth. When family relationships become distant or dysfunctional, many people create substitute families in the form of close friends. In later life, these close friendships can provide the emotional, social, and caregiving support that families are not providing because of emotional or geographical distance.

Generally, older people are isolated from their families only if they choose to be, or if they are so frail or impaired that they cannot reach out and function as social beings. Studies show that family ties are the norm in later life, and that close bonds tend to persist. Some of these bonds are based on love, and some on filial responsibility, a sense of personal obligation that adult children feel toward their aging parents (Schaie & Willis, 2002). But even when bonds are close, times of conflict alternate with times of relative harmony. This seems to be the norm rather than the exception.

## HISTORICAL PERSPECTIVES ON THE FAMILY

It is difficult to fully grasp the older person's perspective on family relationships without acknowledging the importance of their history. This means acquiring an understanding of family dynamics for the period from approximately 1950 to 1980, the postwar era of relative prosperity, when the present population of elderly people married and raised their children. This period was marked by a belief in traditional "family values," defined as desirable and important goals that serve as guiding principles for maintaining one's family (Blanchard-Fields, Hertzog, Stein, & Pak, 2001). This was exemplified by the television portrayal of harmonious, seemingly well-adjusted families on programs such as "Father Knows Best" and "Leave It to Beaver." Family problems such as parent–child conflicts, sibling conflicts, divorce, and illegitimacy were thought of as exceptions to the norm.

Many changes in the family have occurred since the 1950s. People are marrying later or deciding not to marry; birth rates have declined dramatically; many more women are in the work force; divorce rates have tripled; single-parent families have increased dramatically; out-of-wedlock births have increased; and homosexual couples have become more public, often making decisions to have or adopt children. As a result of these changes, the traditional family model—the husband as breadwinner and the wife as homemaker—makes up only about 7% of all U.S. families (Duxbury & Higgins, 1991).

The historical period in which the present older generation was socialized promoted traditional family values. As a result, many older people view these changes as detrimental and as an indication that the family is falling apart. Older generations have been found to be more conservative with respect to women's rights, issues of marriage, and sexual practices (Troll & Skaff, 1997). Others have acknowledged and accepted these changes, and even applauded them as positive.

The baby boomers, the next cohort of older people, were raised by this generation, and therefore were somewhat influenced by their values. However, this upcoming older group has also been influenced by shifting value and role structures, including more openness to social change in which variability of norms is the norm. The "free-spirit" influence of the 1960s and 1970s has changed many of their expectations regarding traditional family values, accepting diverse family styles, and limiting judgmental attitudes. Some now middle-aged and older individuals were influenced by the "me generation" movement of the 1970s, incorporating intimacy-at-a-distance and fleeing from commitment in their personal and family relationships (Tepper, 1994). However, intimacy-at-a-distance has become a more common reaction to older parents, whereby regular, supportive, and affectionate bonds remain, but most contact is not in person, but by telephone or e-mail.

## PARENT–CHILD RELATIONSHIPS

Family relationships in later life were realistically studied and described by Silverstone and Hyman (1976) at the Benjamin Rusk Institute in Cleveland, Ohio. They identified several issues that were found to greatly influence the relationship between the elderly and their adult children. The first of these issues requires the adult child to face up to feelings regarding their aging, perhaps frail parents. The realization that there is a need to provide assistance to aging parents should draw attention to the question of why help is given. The identification of constraints and barriers that may make caregiving difficult needs to be discussed openly. Feelings are rarely consistent, and that fact needs to be acknowledged. Positive feelings such as love, compassion, respect, and tenderness are often experienced alongside some negative feelings such as indifference, fear, anxiety, anger, hostility, contempt, and shame. The combination of these opposing feelings can lead adult children to behaviors such as denial and withdrawal, which, of course, can be counterproductive, and can influence both quality and quantity of time spent with parents.

The second issue requires the adult child to accept his or her parents' old age. The often-hidden emotion of anger can surface and present additional conflict for the adult child. This is closely related to the third issue: namely, that the adult children need to realistically accept their own aging. The acceptance of our own mortality and our feelings about old people certainly influence our attitudes about our own aging. Those who accept their own mortality, feel positive about older people, and have positive attitudes toward aging are more likely to be able to reach out to their elderly parents. The frailty and eventual death of parents represent the symbolic loss of shelter and protection, even when shelter and protection are no longer necessary. The fourth issue requires adult children to acknowledge whether or not they like their aging parents. This is closely related to feelings that go beyond social expectations of "honoring thy father and thy mother" and general expectations of duty. The fifth issue requires the adult child to accept a different status. This new status often results in a reversed dependency relationship, and the acknowledgment of parents' weakness, loss of power, and loss of their parental role. The feelings produced by this role change include resentment, anger, fear, and sadness.

The sixth issue for the adult child is guilt. The potentially overwhelming feeling of guilt resulting from all of the above issues can lead to lowered self-esteem and even a subconscious wish for punishment. Unresolved or unacknowledged feelings can cause a variety of behaviors that are often counterproductive in the relationship between adult children and their aging parents. Some of these behaviors are withdrawal, oversolicitousness, domination, faultfinding, denial, outmoded role playing, protracted adolescent rebellion, blind overinvolvement, and scapegoating (Silverstone & Hyman, 1976).

A partial answer to the challenges raised by some of these issues and the resultant feelings and behaviors these issues elicit is the communication of feelings. Families often talk *at* each other instead of *with* each other. This may have always been their family style. Adult children need to communicate feelings to each other as well as to their parents; older people also need to open communication lines to their adult children. There is often a need for families to have "forums" or "roundtables" where all concerned are present and feelings can be expressed without fear of consequences. Short-term family counseling can facilitate this goal, and will be discussed in a later chapter.

Adult children's behavior and attitudes are often shaped by their parents' behavior. Parents may employ manipulation to get what they want. Denial of infirmities involves pretending that no problems exist and that all is well (this is often used to prevent placement into a long-term-care facility). The exaggeration of infirmities involves the exploitation of their age (this is often done as a play for sympathy, a demand for attention, and/or a request for help). Self-belittlement involves putting themselves down for the purpose of receiving positive and supportive feedback. Money-related behaviors are often used to control family members, especially in families where money is equated with love and where withholding money is equated with withholding of love. Unfortunately, adult children may react to these behaviors by withdrawal or extreme stress responses. But understanding that these behaviors are often a cry for attention and assistance may mobilize the family into action on behalf of the older family member. On the other hand, it has been the experience of the author that occasionally it can be the adult child who is responsible for some of the behavior and attitudes of the older person. Presumably well-meaning family members often consider the older person incapable of dealing with life decisions. This attitude can lead to forced dependence and a self-fulfilling prophecy of helplessness.

## GRANDPARENTHOOD

One of the most delightful role transitions in life is the stage at which parents become grandparents. It is an exciting period of time for most adults, as it brings new challenges with new opportunities (Tepper, 1994). Based on historical stereotypes, society has created an image of grandparents as gray-haired, passive, angelic types, with not much else to do than to be grandparents. However, twenty-first-century grandparents are dispelling that myth in a variety of ways. They are finding themselves balancing multiple roles and possible role conflicts. Typically, they are still employed, married, and possibly have living parents who now require their caregiving attention (Szinovacz, 1998).

Several themes emerge when the meaning of grandparenting and the behaviors involved are analyzed. First, a wide variety of individual styles of grandparenting exist. These are closely related to and influenced by such factors as the gender, age, ethnic background, personality, and financial status of the grandparent. Bengtson and Robertson (1985) have identified a variety of symbolic functions fulfilled by grandparents. Grandparents provide stability, are considered to be an emergency resource, often negotiate between generations, and are useful for constructing the family biography.

One of the most important roles of contemporary grandparents is the transmission of values, morals, and family traditions. Although parents have this major responsibility, parent–child conflicts may influence their acceptance, thereby putting grandparents in a positive position to influence grandchildren in a way that parents may find difficult. From the period of 1970 to 2000, the number of single mothers increased from 3 million to 10 million (U.S. Bureau of the Census, 2001). This dramatic shift in family style has resulted in many grandparents assisting with the raising of their grandchildren.

Neugarten and Weinstein (1964) have identified five styles of grandparenting, three of which are traditional and two more contemporary. Traditional roles were labeled "formal": those who leave the parenting to the parents, but like to offer special favors to the grandchild; the "surrogate parent," usually the grandmother, who assumes parental responsibilities for the child (at the request of the parent); and the "reservoir of family wisdom," usually the grandfather, who maintains his authority and sees himself as the provider of special skills or knowledge. Two more contemporary roles have emerged that tend to be characteristic of younger grandparents. They include the "fun-seeker," who tends to ignore authority issues and often joins the child in enjoyable activities, and the "distant figure," who has only brief and fleeting contact with the grandchild, and is present only at special occasions. These roles hold true into the twenty-first century and continue to be studied aspects of grandparenting (Silverstein & Marenco, 2001).

Because approximately half of all marriages end in divorce, there are many older people with divorced children. This can strongly affect their relationship with grandchildren, as visitation rights can be nonexistent. This is especially true when the divorced child happens to be a son, as mothers get custody in 90% of divorce settlements. However, both sons- and daughters-in-law have the potential to sever ties with their former in-laws, causing a great deal of emotional pain and anger. Several states have enacted grandparent-rights statutes whereby grandparents can petition for visitation. On the positive side, however, grandparents can indeed fill an emotional void created in the lives of children of divorced or separated parents. They can provide consistency, continuity, and a sense of security to their grandchildren.

Because increasing numbers of people are living into very old age, there is a rapidly rising number of great-grandparents. Most of these are women who married at a relatively young age and had children and grandchildren who did the same. Depending on the age of the great-grandparent, great-grandparenthood can bring either intense satisfaction or great frustration. Often great-grandparents experience a greater amount of disability and related health problems. On the other hand, being a great-grandparent can provide an individual with a great sense of personal achievement and family renewal, reaffirming personal generativity and the continuance of their family lines. Knowing that their family will live beyond their own lifetime can be a source of comfort that may help older people face death. The sense that one has lived long enough to produce a fourth generation is a source of status and a mark of distinction to many older people.

## NON-GRANDPARENTING

Non-grandparenting has become an alternative to traditional grandparent expectations for many older adults. A growing number of adults are deciding not to marry, and many married people are deciding not to have children, due to both dual-career lifestyles and personal choice. Some have decided to have children later, possibly as late as their forties. This may be a source of disappointment for those older people expecting and looking forward to grandparenthood. Feelings of deprivation, betrayal, confusion, disappointment, and even anger at their children's life-choice decisions can become a source of stress. Dealing with these strong emotions without having them negatively influence the quality of their relationships with their children can be difficult (Tepper, 1994).

## MARRIAGE

For many older people, marriages of forty or more years have become much more common due largely to rising life expectancy. Older people need love, affection, and social interaction just as do people of all ages. Extensive research has been conducted on marital satisfaction, but not much data have been collected on long-term marriages. Overall marital satisfaction has been measured highest at the beginning of marriage, falls gradually until the children leave home, and rises again in later life (Berry & Williams, 1987). Marital satisfaction has been known to be lowest in midlife, but satisfaction usually begins to rebound when adult children are launched, also known as the "empty nest" period. This improvement is largely due to increased financial resources, relief from daily parenting duties, and the additional time that husbands and wives have together (Cavanaugh, 1997). Marital satisfaction among older couples rises shortly after retirement, but decreases as health problems and age increase. Critical factors that are related to marital problems vs. marital satisfactions in later life include, but are not limited to, discrepant rates of aging and health status, narcissism, fear of death, and the older couple's relationship to children and grandchildren (Lee, 1988).

Many of the long-term marriages we see today are the result of stable relationships characterized by intimacy and close friendship. However, some may become stressful and even dysfunctional as a result of shifts in roles for each partner. Many of the current 40-or-more-year marriages are experiencing a relatively new phenomenon: retirement. Pre-retirement years saw couples busy with child rearing, work, and a strong desire to spend more time together. If the retirement years are not well planned in advance, the partners may find that they are on a prolonged vacation, with limitless amounts of time together. Formerly working couples now find themselves at home for most of their day; women who were homemakers with set routines may now have their husbands "underfoot" all day, as they continue many of their established household routines. Some women may resent their husband's newfound life of leisure, disturbed by the fact that their work continues as usual, without assistance or cooperation from their spouse.

## DIVORCE

Older couples in long-term marriages are less likely to divorce due to disagreements concerning relatively minor issues than are younger couples. They may have different criteria for marital satisfaction, which also may contribute to the low divorce rate among this population (Tepper, 1994). Many have witnessed divorce among their own children and grandchildren, and this has brought most of them great sadness. Some older couples may use this experience to reevaluate their own marriages, and even to seek divorce because of the increased social acceptance of this decision. Caregiving to a sick spouse is an additional source of stress, and often results in the healthy spouse's being torn between the desire to provide care and the need to have a life with activities and friends outside this role. If partners do not share interests and hobbies, and/or have their own interests apart from each other, the possibility of friction exists. Financial strain may occur if their lifestyle must be altered because less discretionary money is available to spend. The average couple will spend as many as 20 years or more in retirement, and so lack of advance preparation can bring about conflict, anger, depression, and apathy. Even with advance preparation, some couples have difficulty in their long-term marriages. Some of these couples had a marital style of quarreling, and continue their battles into later life. Some have had periodic separations or thoughts of divorce, but have remained together because of their reliance and dependence on each other, as well as their history of shared experiences. Generally, however, strong bonds have been formed, and beneath the anger and quarreling is a close attachment.

## SEXUALITY

Society's stereotypes of an asexual old age remain pervasive, shaping popular images of older people and adding to a self-fulfilling prophesy. Gott and Hinchliff (2003) examined how sex is prioritized in middle age and later life. Participants who did not consider sex to be of any importance had neither a current sexual partner, nor felt they would have another partner in their lifetime. However, all participants who had a current partner rated sex as somewhat important, with many rating sex as very or extremely important. Barriers to being sexually active led some to place less importance on sex, especially those who were widowed and those with health problems.

The American Association of Retired Persons Sexuality Study (1999) provided an abundant amount of information about sexual activity and attitudes of adults 45 and over. Although frequency of sexual intercourse declined from age 45 to 85 from 55% to 19% of males and from 50% to 7% of females, other types of sexual activity were reported for both groups, including sexual touching, kissing, and hugging. Oral sexual activity was reported in both males and females, as was self-stimulation in all study groups.

A six-year study of people between 46 and 70 years of age revealed that sexuality remained important for a majority of the respondents, although nearly all reported a decline in their sexual interest and activity. Women attributed the end of their sexual relationships to their husbands (caused by spouse's death, divorce, illness, or inability to perform sexually); men who felt responsible for stopping sexual relations attributed it to inability to perform, loss of interest in sex, or illness. The most significant factor contributing to present sexual activity was past enjoyment of sexuality. Sexual activity generally remained relatively stable among those couples who enjoyed sexual relations in their younger years. But if it did cease, it was due predominantly to changes in health rather than other factors (George & Weiler, 1981; Pfeiffer & Davis, 1974). Research by Starr and Weiner (1981) found a high degree of interest in sexuality and sexual activity. Many in fact reported that sex was as satisfying as or even more satisfying than in earlier years.

Sexual dysfunction in older males is not necessarily caused by age. Masters and Johnson (1970) found six reasons for this phenomenon: (1) monotony of a repetitious sexual relationship, (2) preoccupation with career or economic situations, (3) mental or physical fatigue, (4) overindulgence in food or alcohol, (5) physical or mental infirmities of either the individual or his partner, and (6) fear of performance associated with or resulting from any of the other categories. Other possible causes of dysfunction include high blood pressure, certain types of prostatectomies, uncontrolled diabetes mellitus, side effects of medicine, and depressive episodes. Fear about the effects of sexual exertion on the heart is another concern, often unfounded. Some changes in sexual function are iatrogenic—medically based—or are the result of lack of information about a condition or treatment side effect. When a patient is not informed of possible side effects of medication, is not prepared for surgical side effects, or is told to "take it easy" without further explanation, the result can be sexual problems with concomitant emotional distress. Health care professionals should be aware of the need to discuss these concerns (Thienhaus, 1988).

Intervention strategies for sexual concerns include a medical evaluation that can rule out physical causes of sexual changes, medical treatment if necessary, marital counseling, group or individual counseling, and support groups for those with physical conditions that impact upon sexual attitude or ability (Butler, Lewis, & Sunderland, 1998). Men (13%) are more apt to seek medical attention for sexual dysfunction than women (6%). Since its development, Viagra has become the treatment of choice for males of all ages.

## WIDOWHOOD

It is not surprising that women are much more likely than men to experience the death of a spouse. Widows outnumber widowers by nearly six to one (U.S. Bureau of the Census, 2001). Reasons for this include women's longer life expectancy, the likelihood that women marry older men, and the higher remarriage rate of men.

Losing a spouse causes a major family life transition that requires different levels and kinds of adjustments. It has the potential of creating great distress and forces the individual to cope with the absolute loss of a long-term or often lifelong partner, to adapt to life as a single person, to take on new responsibilities and activities, and possibly to change living arrangements (Tepper, 1994). Options include deciding to live alone; moving in with an adult child, other relative, or single friend; having others move into the now single household; or moving into a residence for older people, thereby increasing the social network and reducing domestic responsibilities (such as cooking, shopping, and cleaning). Whatever the choice, the transition is both difficult and complex and requires a great deal of adaptation during the months or years that follow.

As a result of the higher numbers of widowed females, most of the research on widowhood reflects the widow's rather than the widower's experience. Research on widowers indicates that their major concerns are with unfamiliar domestic and self-maintenance tasks. However, they are more likely to belong to social organizations, to have friends, to drive a car, and to have income higher than their female counterparts (Crandall, 1985). Widowhood appears to affect women less negatively, perhaps because they are able to form close ties with other women (Hatch & Bulcroft, 1992). This is not as true for younger widows, as they have no peer group experience and are typically less prepared. At all ages, loss of a husband often causes financial stress because a major income source is lost (Scannell-Desch, 2003). Recent studies show that widowed persons had higher levels of informal social participation (telephone contact, socializing with friends) than nonwidowed persons, whereas formal social participation (religious participation, meeting attendance, volunteer obligations) levels were comparable between the two groups. Social participation decreases before the death of a spouse, primarily because of poor spousal health and caregiving responsibilities. However, it generally increases following the loss because of increased support from friends and relatives (Utz, Carr, Nesse, & Wortman, 2002). Implications are such that maintaining continuity in the area of social participation is a strategy older adults use to cope with spousal loss. However, not all widowed persons have the same resources to alter their levels of social participation.

Lopata (1973) has found three general patterns of adaptation to widowhood for women. The "self-initiating woman" continued relationships with her children, developed relationships that provided personal intimacy, created a lifestyle that suited her needs and potential, and, in general, adapted to match the resources available to further her own needs and goals. A second pattern was the "ethnic woman," living in an ethnic community, who did not experience much change; was involved in relationships with relatives, friends, and neighbors; and generally lived out her life as she was socialized to do. The third group, "social isolates," never had been highly involved in close social relationships. They were unable to maintain their few previous relationships because friends had moved away, died, or excluded them because of their new single status, and these social contacts were not replaced. They also had less money, which influenced their ability to resocialize. More contemporary research on widowhood has found the above to still be valid, but has also shown that there is an increased proportion of "self-initiating women" who develop a new social life with friends, especially if they live in an area with other widows. Higher rates of social involvement outside the home than their married counterparts have also been observed (Utz et al., 2002). However, health problems, loneliness, and financial strains may be major sources of stress for older widows. It has been found that one effect of widowhood is weight loss, eating more meals alone, most of which were commercially prepared and less healthy, and fewer homemade meals. They reported decreased appetite and decreased enjoyment of their meals (Shahar, Schultz, Shahar, & Wing, 2001). Implications for a multidisciplinary assessment and intervention are apparent, and will be discussed further in chapter 16: "Interdisciplinary Teamwork."

## FAMILY CAREGIVING

Just as myths about aging exist in our society, so do myths about the relationships between generations. The belief that families abandon their elderly is false and unfair to the middle generation. The assumption is that caregiving roles are being relinquished by adult children, but, in point of fact, the older population is healthier and more independent than previous cohorts. Those who may need some care may be living with formal assistance in the increasing number of community-based housing facilities for older people that will be discussed in chapter 3: "The Nursing Home and the Continuum of Care."

Providing care to an ill family member is undoubtedly a stressful experience, one that much research has consistently associated with poorer psychological well-being (Bookwala, Yee, & Schulz, 2000). Although the vast amount of caregivers are female and middle-aged, national estimates indicate that up to 25% of caregivers are male, and a sizable number of caregivers (12%–40%) are older adults (National Alliance for Caregiving, 1997). Furthermore, an older spouse is most likely to be the caregiver for an impaired, community-living adult, and spouses are more prevalent among caregivers over age 65 than in other age groups (American Psychological Association, 1997). Caregiving demands and their concomitant links to mental health problems among elderly spouse caregivers are recently demanding attention among researchers, mental health practitioners, social service agencies, health care providers, and public policy planners.

Middle-aged children still assume a considerable number of caregiving functions. Issues related to caregiving are reflected in some of the needs expressed by this middle generation. A primary issue is that of role strains. Who gets their primary allegiance: their family of orientation (their parents) or their family of procreation (their spouse, children, and grandchildren)? Role strain also involves dealing with what is sometimes referred to as the "bereavement overload" of their elderly parents, that devastating sense of grief associated with repeated multiple and irreparable losses. There are three stressful situations that the author has observed over the years that are believed to be the most difficult for caregivers (Tepper, 1994).

The first stressor is bringing a parent into their home. This requires substantial readjustment of the host couple's routine and should include the following considerations before a decision is made. Can the caregiver talk with the parent on a variety of subjects without becoming embarrassed or angry? Does the caregiver's spouse get along with the parent? Has the parent asked to live with the adult child? Would the parent have some privacy in the adult child's home? Could the parent adjust to the caregiver's way of life? Could the parent maintain present friendships while living in the caregiver's home? Would the parent let the adult child be the boss in his or her own home? Could the parent adapt to the adult child's way of cooking? Is the parent able to do simple chores around the house? Could the caregiver avoid overprotecting the parent? And vice versa? Does the caregiver's present income allow for an additional household member? Could the adult child perform the eventual personal care tasks that the parent may need? This decision should not be made without considering other possibilities, such as living with several adult children alternatively, living with the parent's sibling, cousin, niece, or other relative, or relocating to an environment suited specifically to the physical, social, and emotional needs of the older person. The extreme stresses of caregiving require management on the part of the caregiver. This may include self-help or professional assistance (Tepper, 1993).

A second stressor is the decision to place a severely incapacitated parent into a nursing home. The obviously high degree of guilt involved in this decision produces a great deal of stress for adult children. At this point they should consider researching the alternatives to institutional care, such as home health care services, congregate-care adult homes, respite care, day care, community based congregate-meal programs, geriatric mental health programs, legal services, visiting nurse services, chore services, and meals-on-wheels programs. A thorough knowledge of available community services in the long-term-care system may provide viable alternatives to institutional placement.

The crisis of contending with a mentally ill, acting-out, violent parent can also be incredibly stressful. Disorientation, memory loss, confusion, insomnia, and incontinence can wreak havoc on the emotional life of the caregiver. The task at hand is often that of accepting the fact that this is no longer the parent who once existed, as there eventually may be no trace of the personality that was previously known. A multidimensional diagnosis of disturbing behavior is often necessary, taking into account such factors as the onset of symptoms, changes in family health, family expectations, physical condition, recent losses, side effects of medication, stress, the use of alcohol or drugs, and change in family structure, as these may be indicative of reversible conditions that are responsive to treatment. A team of health care specialists consisting of an internist, psychiatrist, audiologist, social worker, psychologist, neurologist, and radiologist may be necessary to assist in diagnosing these conditions. Further discussion will take place in chapter 9: "Major Mental Disorders of Old Age."

## DEMENTIA AND THE FAMILY

Mobilizing the family for the purpose of caregiving is often a central issue in family relationships. Two issues that will be explored in chapter

10, "Counseling Older People and their Families," are how to help a family cope with the frustrating, disruptive, and often embarrassing behavior of a person with dementia, and how to help those who do the caregiving find ways to ease the stress, thereby preventing burnout. The author has observed that the amount of burden family members experience caring for a relative with dementia is related to the support they receive from other family members and friends. The primary caregiver benefits from the individual or group counseling to be discussed in chapter 10, but when involving other family members to support the primary caregiver, individual counseling is often not the answer. Families have been known to dissolve close, longstanding ties when dementia caregiving or decisions regarding institutionalization come up. This will also be further discussed in chapter 10.

## CONCLUSION

Developmental issues in later life are inextricably related to and result from family relationships. Older people can best be understood in the context of their families. This chapter has described some of the more common family patterns in later life, demonstrating the complexity of older people's social worlds. Professionals working with older families need to be cognizant of this complexity when assessing situations and planning interventions.

Professionals must recognize the great diversity that exists among elders and among family styles of communication. Older people are individuals with long histories of family interaction; they have roles and relationships that have both changed and remained constant. Families differ in their expectations and the quality of their interactions. Lifestyle differences among older persons, couples, and families need to be addressed before problems can be dealt with. Familiarity with their cultural and ethnic backgrounds will also help professionals understand their preferences. All of these factors will affect their approach to decision making and problem solving, and are important considerations when interventions are proposed.

## REFERENCES

American Association of Retired Persons. (1999). American Association of Retired Persons Sexuality Study. Washington, DC: AARP. Available at www.aarp.org/research/sexuality

American Psychological Association. (1997). *What practitioners should know about working with older adults.* Washington, DC: Author.

Bengtson, V. L., & Robertson, I. F. (Eds.). (1985). *Grandparenthood.* Beverly Hills, CA: Sage.

Berry, R. E., & Williams, F. L. (1987). Assessing the relationship between quality of life and marital and income satisfaction. *Journal of Marriage and the Family, 49,* 107–116.

Blanchard-Fields, F., Hertzog, C., Stein, R., & Pak, R. (2001). Beyond a stereotyped view of older adults' traditional family values. *Psychology and Aging, 16*(3), 483–496.

Bookwala, J., Yee, J. L., & Schultz, R. (2000). Caregiving and detrimental mental and physical health outcomes. In G. M. Williamson, P. A. Parmelee, & D. R. Schaffer (Eds.), *Physical illness and depression in older adults: A handbook of theory, research, and practice* (pp. 93–131). New York: Plenum.

Butler, R. N., Lewis, M., & Sunderland, T. (1998). *Aging and mental health.* New York: Allyn & Bacon.

Cavanaugh, J. C. (1997). *Adult development and aging.* Boston: Brooks-Cole.

Crandall, R. (1985). *Gerontology: A behavioral science approach.* Reading, MA: Addison-Wesley.

Duxbury, L. E., & Higgins, C. A. (1991). Gender differences in work-family conflict. *Journal of Applied Psychology, 76,* 60–73.

George, L. K., & Weiler, S. J. (1981). Sexuality in middle and later life: The effects of age, cohort, and gender. *Archives of General Psychiatry, 38,* 919–923.

Gott, M., & Hinchliff, S. (2003). How important is sex in later life? The views of older people. *Social Science and Medicine, 56*(8), 1617–1628.

Hatch, L. R., & Bulcroft, K. (1992). Contact with friends in later life: Disentangling the effects of gender and marital status. *Journal of Marriage and the Family, 54,* 222–232.

Lee, A. R. (1988). Kinship and social support of the elderly: The case of the U.S. *Aging and Society, 5,* 19–38.

Lopata, H. Z. (1973a). Support systems of American urban widowhood. *Journal of Gerontological Issues, 44*(3), 113–128.

Masters, W. H., & Johnson, V. E. (1970). *Human sexual inadequacy.* Boston: Little, Brown.

National Alliance for Caregiving. (1997). Family caregiving in the U.S.: Findings from a national survey. Final report. Bethesda, MD: National Alliance for Caregiving.

Neugarten, B. L., & Weinstein, K. K. (1964). The changing American grandparent. *Journal of Marriage and the Family, 26,* 299–304.

Pfeiffer, E., & Davis, G. (1974). Determinants of sexual behavior in middle age and old age. In E. Palmore (Ed.), *Normal aging 2: Reports of the Duke longitudinal study, 1970–1973* (pp. 251–252). Durham, NC: Duke University Press.

Scannell-Desch, E. (2003). Women's adjustment to widowhood. *Journal of Psychosocial Nursing and Mental Health Services, 41*(5), 28–36.

Schaie, K. W., & Willis, S. K. (2002). *Adult development and aging.* Upper Saddle River, NJ: Prentice Hall.

Shahar, D. R., Schultz, R., Shahar, A., & Wing, R. R. (2001). The effect of widowhood on weight change, dietary intake, and eating behavior in the elderly. *Journal of Aging and Health, 13*(2), 189–199.

Silverstein, M., & Marenco, A. (2001). How Americans enact the grandparent role across the family life course. *Journal of Family Issues, 22,* 493–522.

Silverstone, B., & Hyman, H. K. (1976). *You and your aging parent.* New York: Pantheon.

Starr, B. D., & Weiner, M. B. (1981). *The Starr-Weiner report on sex and sexuality in the mature years.* Briarcliff Manor, NY: Stein & Day.

Szinovacz, M. E. (1998). Grandparents today: A demographic profile. *Gerontologist, 38,* 37–52.

Tepper, L. M. (1993a). A life-style rehabilitation approach to manage the stress of caregiving. In L. Tepper & J. Toner (Eds.), *Respite care: Programs, problems, and solutions* (pp. 157–165). New York: Charles.

Tepper, L. M. (1994). Family relationships in later life. In I. Gutheil (Ed.), *Work with older people* (pp. 42–62). New York: Fordham University Press.

Thienhaus, O. J. (1988). Practical overview of sexual function and advancing age. *Geriatrics, 43,* 63–67.

Troll, L. E., & Skaff, M. M. (1997). Perceived continuity of self in old age. *Psychology and Aging, 12,* 162–169.

U.S. Bureau of the Census. (2001). *Current population survey: Households by type, 1970–2000.* Washington, DC: U.S. Government Printing Office.

Utz, R. L., Carr, D., Nesse, R., & Wortman, C. B. (2002). The effect of widowhood on older adults' social participation: An evaluation activity. *Gerontologist, 42*(4), 522–533.

# 3

# The Nursing Home and the Continuum of Care

## William T. Smith

Nursing homes continue to play an important role in the continuum of care and to be a resource to the community at large. They have evolved in response to the needs of their residents and the demands of their community. Throughout much of recorded history seniors resided within the family setting. As they outlived their immediate and/or extended family, or began to demonstrate dementia or other conditions that exceeded the care capability of the family, another setting became necessary. This chapter presents an overview of long-term residential care, beginning with nursing homes and ending with a discussion of the continuum of other housing options available to people as they age.

### THIS HISTORY OF LONG TERM CARE

Nursing homes can trace their history back to the days of the "asylums." Congregate settings became more apparent in communities in response to the aging conditions of individuals. Medical science had not significantly developed in diagnosis and treatment of older persons, who were afflicted with physical and mental conditions preventing them from living independently or harmoniously with other family members. Facilities that housed older persons included lunatic hospitals, lunatic asylums, asylums for the insane, state hospitals, mental health centers, psychiatric hospitals, regional centers, retreats, sanitariums, and developmental centers (Long et al., 2003). In the late 1850s we witnessed the beginning of congregate care facilities, known as homes for the aging. Seniors sought this type of housing as their health needs increased or as they found living with family members no longer an option. In some cases seniors outlived other relatives, making the choice of a congregate living arrangement a suitable option.

For many years the home for the aging, largely occupied by women, was the only evidence of housing for the frail elderly. Many of the homes were developed by churches or fraternal organizations. Residents who became too sick for such congregate living were likely to be placed in a hospital or infirmary. But as infirmaries and hospitals were re-engineered in the late 1800s to respond to advances in medicine and community needs and desires, custodial care for the elderly in this setting was no longer appropriate.

With the onset of Medicare and Medicaid in 1965 the proliferation of nursing homes began. Federal and state governments recognized that demographics were demanding a new environment to serve seniors with chronic disabilities or in need of custodial care and to relieve the burden of hospitals maintaining seniors within their facilities despite their no longer needing acute care services. Federal capital and operational resources were now available and nursing homes were developed in communities around the country.

The nursing home continues to evolve today, from a home for the aged, which provided long-term care and was a last residence for seniors before dying, to a short-term, rehabilitative service prior to returning to community. Initially nursing homes were noted for custodial care and were largely paternalistic in their underlying value base. Common was the practice of regulating the life and supplying or meeting the needs of its residents in a way that is suggestive of a father handling his children. Today other values such as autonomy and choice have replaced a paternalistic approach to providing care.

Federal and state authorities required compliance with regulations in order for facilities to continue within the Medicare/Medicaid program. Prescribed ways of constructing, remodeling, and maintaining nursing homes and the type of services permitted in this level of care were mandated. The federal regulations set the minimum requirements or regulations for participation in the Medicare/Medicaid programs. States have the additional authority to place additional regulations on providers. There is a federal requirement that facilities be "inspected annually." This inspection function has been delegated to the state's department of health, which hires and trains surveyors, who visit the facility, determine compliance, and then completes a report on their findings that is sent to the federal government. States are funded by the federal government to perform this inspection function, but may be audited by the federal government through a "look behind survey." This survey determines if the state surveyors have done an adequate survey or not. It is not unusual for a facility to be surveyed and re-surveyed. The purpose of this is to ensure that states were consistently evaluating nursing homes for continued participation in the Medicare/ Medicaid program.

In recent years provider groups and academics have been attempting to adjust the annual survey requirements by Centers for Medicaid and Medicare Services (CMS) to include a more comprehensive view of nursing home quality with an emphasis on quality of life measures (Kane, 2003).

## QUALITY INDICATORS

Much work has been done to develop quality indicators to help inform a continuous quality improvement program in all nursing homes. Clinical guidelines have been addressed by multidisciplinary groups of profes- sionals to determine the best practice models for nursing homes. There is much discussion about "quality" and what should be the expected and measurable "quality outcomes" in a nursing home. It appears cer- tain that the federal government and the states that conduct the annual surveys will rely on quality indicators as part of a newer system for monitoring and regulating nursing homes (Manard, 2002). Quality indicators are objective measures that evolve through evaluation of procedures employed by practitioners and deemed by experts to be the appropriate way in which care is to be delivered. These indicators are adjusted based on new medical discoveries, or through best practices that professionals refine in meeting the needs of older persons.

The annual survey in a nursing home is very stressful for the staff. A team of inspectors monitoring their daily work; reviewing medical records; interviewing residents, family members, administrators, and key staff; and only citing or reporting negative outcomes, although necessary, can be and often is demoralizing. Even if a facility receives a report at the end of a survey in which no deficiencies are found, these reports are not accompanied with positive commentary. The surveyor's role is to evaluate compliance with federal/state regulations, not to compliment best practices. On the other hand, a report of deficiencies is usually conditional upon a final review. The list of deficiencies must have a plan of correction returned within ten days, and the home may be subject to monetary penalties, a ban on admission, and possible expulsion from the Medicaid and Medicare program unless all conditions are brought back into compliance within a specified time period.

The survey is not an exact science. Interpretation of the federal requirements, measurement of compliance, and consistency from state to state in reporting deficiencies confuse the discussion as to whether nursing homes are more or less compliant with federal regulations (U.S. Department of Health and Human Services, 2003).

## PUBLIC PERCEPTIONS OF CARE FACILITIES

The perception of the public and the government is that far too many nursing homes are having serious quality problems. Daily opportunities for negative situations with frail elderly residents who are dependent on multiple staff contacts or interactions are a reality. This potential for negativity is not an excuse for poor quality care, but rather should be seen as a reason to address the culture of an organization dedicated to caring for frail individuals in a nursing home environment. Even one serious negative quality outcome is too many. Nursing homes should be operated and evaluated in a zero tolerance environment, as far as quality outcome and compliance with regulations are concerned.

The number of nursing homes with serious quality problems remains unacceptably high, despite a decline in the incidence of such reported problems as actual harm or other serious deficiencies. These were cited in 20% or 3,500 nursing homes during an 18-month period ending in January 2002, compared to 29% for an earlier period. This General Accounting report continues with criticism of the survey process at both the state and federal levels (General Accounting Office, 2003).

Among other complex elements of the nursing home, sensitivity to the cultural background of both the resident and the staff has to be addressed. Staff training and educational training for family members together with staff can be a very effective way of improving communication while clarifying expectations from the staff's and family's perspectives.

## THE PARTNERS IN CAREGIVING PROJECT

Institutional life can cause problems for families and sometimes decreases their involvement as a result. In particular, staff–family relations can be strained and conflictual. Nursing home staff are struggling to make ends meet and to provide good care under demanding work conditions. The Partners in Caregiving Project, developed by Karl Pillemer of the Cornell Gerontology Research Institute, is an example of an educational program that aims to meet the needs of both staff and family. It was field tested by the Foundation for Long Term Care (Albany, NY) and implemented as a training program for a large subset of not for profit nursing homes in New York state. This program is an excellent tool for obtaining a better understanding of the respective roles of all concerned.

The program consists of two parallel workshop series: one for family members and one for nursing home staff. Skills such as clear and respectful communication and consideration of cultural and ethnic differences of both groups are developed. Values and approaches for handling blame, criticism, and conflict are stressed. The program concludes with a joint session of staff and family. This comprehensive program has had positive results during the last five years. New and seasoned administrators would benefit by supporting this program within their facility (Pillemer, Hegeman, Dean, Albright, & Meador, 1997).

## EXPANDING THE ROLE OF NURSING HOMES

The nursing home today provides much more than custodial care to its residents. Long-term stay is still prevalent but some residents are now using this setting for short-term stays, subacute stays, rehabilitation, respite care, and palliative care.

Reimbursement systems that evolved since the 1980s have encouraged providers to change the way they use their facilities. Complex reimbursement schemes have developed from state to state, utilizing federal resources, supplemented with state and local reimbursement. Many nursing homes have become expert in providing rehabilitative services through occupational therapy, physical therapy, and speech pathology, along with skilled nursing, dietary specialties, recreational therapy, and social services. All of these services are provided under specific medical orders, with the goal of returning residents to functioning at their highest possible level. Often, the goal is to discharge the resident back into the community.

Some states have developed their Medicaid reimbursement program to be sensitive to "Resource Utilization Groupings" or RUGS. In effect, the states will pay a dollar amount that reflects the category of care in which a resident is classified. For example, the highest category of grouping is referred to as "rehabilitation." Residents who are in this grouping are receiving physical and/or occupational therapies, which must be provided by trained professionals or therapists. Residents are seen daily for intensive therapy. As a result of this high level of service, reimbursement is approximately 80% higher than the average daily rate, as compared to a custodial resident who might be classified in a "PA" grouping, one of the lowest groupings, referring to the custodial care that is provided in meeting the physical assistance needs, provided by a non-skilled employee, like a certified nursing attendant. Residents in this lower grouping are reimbursed at approximately 50% of the average daily rate. This category considers the patient's diagnosis and level of care required to meet the individual's needs. Clearly, documentation on the state-approved tools and in the medical chart become critical in this type of payment scheme. The medical record is also the source for the ongoing quality assurance and survey evaluations by state department of health surveyors described above. These assessments are made on a regular basis, no farther apart than every fifteen months, with most facilities undergoing an onsite evaluation within a twelve-month period.

## LONG-TERM CARE

Long-term care refers to the supportive services required by people whose ability to care for themselves has been reduced by a chronic illness or disability, whether physical or mental. The need for long-term care is often measured in terms of the extent to which an individual requires assistance or supervision in performing basic activities of daily living (ADLs), such as bathing, dressing, toileting, or eating, or instrumental activities of daily living (IADLs), such as meal preparation or managing money. Although most current spending for long-term care is for individuals in nursing homes, the majority of those requiring personal assistance live in the community (Merliss, 1999). Home care will be discussed in depth in a subsequent chapter.

### Financing Long Term Care

Although the financing of care for the elderly will be discussed in depth in chapter 12, "Financing Health Care," it is important to provide the reader with preliminary financial information related to long-term care. Medicaid is the major third-party payer for nursing home care, whereas Medicare has emerged as the largest single payer for home care. Combined, the two programs pay for 56% of nursing home and home health care. Most of the remaining costs are paid by the individual or by family savings (Merliss, 1999).

Medicaid is the federal–state program of medical assistance for certain groups of the poor, including families with children, the elderly, and the disabled. Medicare is a federally funded program, which reimburses providers in certain medical situations where there is evidence that rehabilitation or skilled nursing services can be employed for no more than one hundred days for each spell of illness, resulting in the patient regaining independence or improved functioning as a result of this trained intervention. Examples of this type of service would be a physical therapist working with a patient after fracturing a hip, who receives therapy and learns how to ambulate again. Another example would be a patient having an open wound, who received skilled nursing treatment accompanied with medication, which heals the wound. Ordinarily, people qualify for this program by meeting limits on both their income and their assets. Most states also allow the "medically needy," or those with large medical bills to elect to reduce (give back) their income levels to qualify for Medicaid. There is also a provision called "spending down," which allows individuals to reduce their assets by paying for their care until their assets have been reduced to the state's limit (Merliss, 1999).

Nursing home care is very expensive and may amount to over $100,000 per year. As a result, only a small percentage of elderly are paying privately, and many of those are only in that status during a spend-down period. Private insurance, long-term care insurance, and managed care are considered small payers, but may be looked upon in the future to support this level of care if the insurance product changes to attract greater use by the elderly and by healthy younger adults.

## The Determination of Payment Rate: The Prospective Rate System

With the Balanced Budget Act (BBA) of 1997 payment for Medicare skilled nursing facility (SNF) services moved to a "prospective payment" system. Effective with cost reporting periods beginning on or after July 1, 1998, skilled nursing facilities were no longer paid on a reasonable cost basis or through low volume prospectively determined rates, but rather on the basis of a prospective payment system (PPS). The PPS payment rate is adjusted for case mix (the average amount of care necessary for all patients) and geographic variation in wages. This rate covers all costs of providing covered SNF services (routine, ancillary, and capital-related costs) (Centers for Medicare & Medicaid Services, 2003).

With the prospective payment system came a need for operators of nursing homes to become better informed on cost accounting and uncovering the information necessary to fill out cost reports. Finance departments became more sophisticated, and for the past twenty years have become more dependent on computer and technological advances to ensure that maximum reimbursement was obtained. Managers within departments were educated on the need for proper budgeting. The use of computers, intellectual technology, and data analysis is spreading into program areas and becoming linked to fiscal data sites to ensure effective financial management of the total organization.

It soon became recognized that staffing and employee-related expenses such as benefits are the largest area of cost within the nursing home. Many of these cost centers exploded as labor unions began to organize this work force, driving up hourly wages, and improving benefits such as overtime enhancement, shift differentials, vacation and holiday time, and medical insurance.

## THE GROWTH OF LONG-TERM INSTITUTIONAL CARE

There are approximately 1.56 million seniors living in nursing homes. This number represents 4.5% of Americans over 65 years of age. The percentage changes dramatically when analyzed by age: 1.1% are between 65 and 74 years of age; 4.7% are 75 to 84 years of age; and 1.8% are 85+ years of age (U.S. Administration on Aging, 2003).

Of the 17,000 nursing homes in the country in 2000, approximately 25% or 4,250 were nonprofit or governmental sponsored, with the remaining homes (75% or 12,750) identified as proprietary or for profit. Many of the latter group are owned and operated by alliances or Wall Street chains, organized under private ownership, and may distribute profits or surplus to stockholders or investors. The nonprofit sponsors, many of which where originally sponsored by faith and fraternal based organizations, do not distribute year end surpluses but rather use the surpluses, if any, within the corporation or to develop new programs for seniors (U.S. Administration on Aging, 2003).

According to the National Center for Health Statistics, the trend in nursing home size has changed over the past thirty years. There has been a decrease in the number of smaller facilities, those with fewer than fifty residents. In 1973 this group of small facilities amounted to 41% of all nursing homes in the United States. By the year 2000 only

11.5% of nursing homes were categorized as small. During this same time period those nursing homes having between fifty and ninety-nine residents continued to average about 35–39% of homes. The number of larger homes, those with between 100 and 200 residents doubled, from 20% in 1973 to 42% in 2000. There was also a doubling of the largest nursing homes, those with over 200 residents, from 4% to 8% (National Center for Health Statistics, 2002).

In the 1970s it was also common to see hospitals building their own nursing homes and establishing them as hospital-based or free-standing facilities. The new facilities allowed hospitals to move patients out of acute care areas to either lighter-staffed units or into specific facilities for the skilled nursing resident, allowing the hospitals to utilize their beds for higher intensity-of-care patients, and frequently higher reimbursed patients than those who were rehabilitating or who needed custodial care.

It is apparent that the era of the "mom and pop" nursing home is coming to a close. The complexity of operating a nursing home and the level of care required discourages the smaller facility from remaining in the business of providing care. The law of numbers has come into play, and smaller nursing homes have been urged either to grow or align themselves with larger organizations. There also seems to be a trend for private nursing homes to care for two hundred or fewer residents, whereas the larger nursing homes generally are operated by nonprofit sponsors.

## WORK FORCE ISSUES

The staff of any long-term care facility plays a critical role in producing quality outcomes. The role of direct-care workers has been found to have a profound influence on the debate about what constitutes quality care (Stone, 2003). It is the direct-care staff, not the nurses or doctors, that provide eight out of every ten hours of care that residents receive (McDonald, 1994). The central importance of human interaction in a long-term care facility is one of the major reasons work force development should be considered an important element of defining and measuring quality. The sensitive areas of the daily routines of caring for residents requires that the staff be skilled and prepared to deal with personal interaction issues.

It is critical for the administrator or operator to have an understanding of the motivators that recruit and retain employees. Not surprisingly, compensation is a key element in determining whether someone will accept employment. However, several studies of turnover have singled out the relationship between direct-care workers and supervisors as a significant factor in job retention (Bowers et al., 2003).

The development of the work force is not adequately viewed as a priority either from the regulatory perspective or in the development and implementation of quality improvement initiatives. Stone (2003) believes that a number of factors contribute to this situation: (1) providers lack motivation to invest in their work force, (2) economic, racial, and ethnic differences exist between workers and employers, (3) there is a hidden nature to the relationship between clients and workers, (4) workers lack a voice, (5) the regulatory system is not designed to address work force issues, and (6) human resource management expertise and models of successful work force development are limited. Many researchers in this field have indicated that a nursing home can be judged by the relationship between the Administrator and the Director of Nursing Service. If there was synergy between the two, there seemed to be a correlation with high resident and family satisfaction as well as positive results on annual state and federal inspections. Although this relationship remains critical, researchers have begun to delve more deeply in their analysis of work force issues and have looked at other relationships within the organization.

The paraprofessional long-term care work force—nurse aides, home health and home care aides, personal care workers, and personal care attendants—forms the nucleus of the formal long-term care system. Nationally, there are approximately two million direct care workers providing hands-on care, supervision, and emotional support to millions of elderly and younger people with chronic illnesses and disabilities. Providers and state agencies responsible for long-term care are reporting unprecedented vacancies and turnover among direct care workers. National data show annual turnover rates ranging from about 45 percent to over 100 percent for nursing homes (General Accounting Office, 2001).

## Recruitment and Retention

Researchers have studied recruitment and retention practices and have worked with providers to determine effective ways to help reduce high vacancy and turnover rates among direct care staff. There is also a growing awareness that the work force pool may be shrinking due to an increase in older persons in our society, and a reduced birthrate resulting in fewer workers to meet the needs of an increasing number of older persons. This shift in demographics compounds an already difficult situation. A California study looked at wages and benefits and found that caregiver occupations fare less well than competing occupations in terms of wages, benefits, and opportunities for advancement. Occupations in the same labor market that are similar to nurses aide work offer 10% higher wages (Ong, Rickles, Matthias, & Benjamin, 2002). Over 70% of the respondents in another study believed that the cause of their recruitment problems is better pay in other industries (Stone, 2003).

## Management Issues in Quality Care

Nursing home operators today need to be more aware of the types of supervisory skills of their managers. Nursing homes typically hire "charge nurses" based on their clinical skills, place them on units to oversee and provide the clinical care, and further expect them to supervise other nurses and direct care workers. Many charge nurses are not trained supervisors. Stone's (2003) study found that whereas direct care workers view charge nurses as supervisors, charge nurses see themselves primarily as clinicians. They do not identify themselves as managers. This is but one example of administration's belief that a supervisory function is in place when in reality it is not. In many nursing schools we find that management and supervision education is limited to one or two courses. Professional health and allied schools of higher education need to enhance their curriculum to respond to this lack.

Promotions to supervisory levels are sometimes based on years of employment. This does not in itself justify promotion to a supervisory level without additional training. It has been found that a major reason employees leave their positions is their relationship with their supervisor. Administrators spend a significant amount of time with their senior management and department heads, but generally expect department heads to manage their own supervisors. The administrator and senior management perceive direct care workers very differently from the way direct care workers perceive themselves (Stone et al., 2003).

There is a growing awareness, however, that the direct care worker has important knowledge of the resident. Managers today are involving direct care workers more with the running of the nursing units and many have permitted direct care workers to participate in the resident care planning process. Incorporating this information in the planning and provision of care has been found to improve the quality outcome for the resident, while raising self-esteem for the direct care worker (Stone et al., 2003).

## Innovative Models of Staff Empowerment

Nursing homes are also seeing new models of staff empowerment that rely on direct care workers using their judgment in time management for accomplishing tasks with the residents. This allows for more creativity in participating with the resident in activities that traditionally would not have been part of their work. Some nursing homes have empowered the staff to handle their scheduling as a team, requiring that the unit be properly staffed, and relying on the team to live within regular pay hours. It then becomes their responsibility to adjust schedules and to accommodate replacement of workers throughout the course of the pay period.

In the interviews conducted as part of the Stone (2003) study, staff members reported that they regarded their workplace like a family. Recruitment and retention problems were reduced and communication and collaboration among the staff were high. Direct care workers were trusted to make decisions affecting resident care and were held accountable. There was improved communication among the direct care worker, the resident, and the family members, resulting in improved overall satisfaction.

The Stone study (2003) identified strategies for expanding the labor pool. There has been recognition that students in elementary and high school need to be introduced to long-term care employment opportunities. All levels of care, including community-based senior service centers, are suitable for internship and volunteer activities. By learning about the role that these settings play within the community, students may consider preparing for a career in the long-term care profession. Other areas that are being explored are the welfare-to-work recipients, men who traditionally do not work in this field, school-to-work students, volunteers, immigrants, and older workers or retirees who are outliving their resources and/or are in need of supplementing their retirement income (Stone, 2003).

## CHANGES IN NURSING HOME UTILIZATION

Residence in a nursing home is an alternative to long-term care provided in one's home or in other community settings (to be discussed later in this chapter). However, recent declines in rates of nursing home residence may reflect broader changes in the health care system, as well as the alternative choices that older people now have. Other forms of residential care and services such as independent housing, supportive housing, assisted living, and home health care have become more prevalent, while rates of nursing home admissions have declined. Declines in disability among the older population may also have contributed to this trend.

In 1997, only 11 per 1,000 people ages 65 to 74 resided in nursing homes, compared with 46 per 1,000 people ages 75 to 84, and 192 per 1,000 ages 85 or older. About half of older nursing home residents in 1997 were 85 or older. The total rate of nursing residence among the older population declined 10% between 1985 and 1997 (Administration on Aging, 2003). The profile of nursing home residents is also changing. They are generally older and sicker, requiring more services to address the diagnoses that they have upon admission. This may be a reflection of the growth of alternative living arrangements that provide a lesser level of care, but care nonetheless.

Many nursing homes have found it difficult to keep their beds occupied. Noting that residents are usually coming into care sicker and more compromised, some nursing home admissions staffs have been cultivating relationships with hospital discharge coordinators. Attempts have been made to admit residents late in the day or even on weekends to accommodate hospital routines and needs. Nursing home staff is marketing directly to doctors and to family members to ensure a smooth transition from the acute care facility to the nursing home. Attempts are being made to educate the community at large on aging issues and wellness concerns. Nursing homes have the opportunity to be hubs of educational information for the community, thereby increasing visibility and improving their image.

Many nursing homes have refined their activities and developed niche areas of expertise that might assist in utilizing their available resources. Dementia care, palliative care, and respite or short stays in the nursing home are becoming more frequent. These will be discussed in greater detail in Part III of this book, as will the broader understanding of adult mortality, an understanding necessary as our country as a whole begins to age in place. The changing causes of death and chronic illness, as well as the prevention of disease and promotion of wellness, will be discussed in Part II.

## HOME- AND COMMUNITY-BASED SERVICE

One reason for the decrease in the use of the nursing home is the increase of Home- and Community-Based Services (HCBS). Most seniors prefer to live independently and within their community. Lifelong networks and relationships gain importance as individuals age. Home- and community-based services will continue to be the major growth area in aging services. Both state and federal governments perceive that moving from institutional services to HCBS will result in less expensive long-term care, and governments are heavily invested in "rebalancing" or "right sizing" the institutional and community-based services mix. Medicaid spending on HCBS increased to 29% of total Medicaid expenditures in fiscal year 2001 from 27% in fiscal year 2000. Legislators understand the strong preference of voters for community-based services. This preference is shared by aging populations and the young disabled (American Association of Homes and Services for the Aging, 2003).

Families of the elderly and the disabled will continue to be the primary sources of caregiving in the community. The informal caregiver is a tremendous resource to the older person. A body of research has been developed detailing the importance of friends and neighbors, spouse, adult children, extended family, and the functionality of informal support systems. The importance of in-kind and volunteer activity would not be affordable by organized and public supports (Cantor, 1979).

Another driver from institutional-based care can be found from a recent Supreme Court decision in the *Olmstead* case, which continues to be a catalyst for increasing HCBS and rebalancing the long-term care systems. Olmstead interpreted the American with Disabilities Act to mean that states must provide services in the most integrated setting appropriate to the needs of individuals with disabilities. The ruling directs states to make "reasonable modifications" in programs and activities. Modifications that would "fundamentally alter" the nature of services, programs or activities, however are not required. As a result of this 1999 Supreme Court ruling, the federal government has encouraged states to plan for reforms not only in the health arena but also in the areas of transportation, housing, education, and other social supports to fully integrate people with disabilities into the least restrictive settings.

Court cases brought under the Americans with Disabilities Act of 1990 generally are decided in favor of plaintiffs, and do not allow states to cut back services or waiver slots, or limit community-based services. For example, a recent decision prohibited Oklahoma from providing fewer prescription medications in HCBS settings than institutional settings. These court cases established a right for individuals to receive services in the least restrictive environment (American Association of Homes and Services, 2003).

Aside from court decisions, there is strong state and federal administrative and legislative support for the philosophy of *Olmstead.* Initial and continuing changes to Medicaid are facilitating transition activity and use of funds for one-time costs related to the transition from the nursing home and home- and community-based services. A total of $160 million (Fiscal Year January 2003) has been appropriated for Real Systems Change Grants, which will be used generally for state HCBS and infrastructure development and nursing home transition programs (American Association of Homes and Services, 2003).

The increase of the older population, their improved health status as a group, and their continued engagement through many activities, volunteerism and work will be additional catalysts for HCBS. Senior Centers throughout the nation, for example, play an important role in keeping the elderly engaged. The social support, educational opportunities, introduction to new roles in later years, and the continued growth of medical science will deter the entry to the nursing home for many baby boomers—the next demographic wave of seniors and policy makers.

## FEDERAL FUNDING FOR KEY AGING PROGRAMS

As of the end of 2003, the budget authority for continuing of Older Americans Act, Title III funding is indicative of a growing preference for home- and community-based services:

| | |
|---|---|
| Supportive Services and Center | $355,673,000 |
| Congregate Meals | $384,592,000 |
| Home Delivered Meals | $180,985,000 |
| USDA Nutrition Program | $148,697,000 |
| Preventive Health Service | $ 21,919,000 |
| Family Caregivers | $149,025,000 |
| Title VII: Vulnerable Older Americans | $ 18,560,000 |
| Alzheimer's Initiative | $ 13,312,000 |

This level of funding is expected to continue and, with the advocacy of constituents, should increase in the years ahead.

## OTHER HOME AND COMMUNITY BASED PROGRAMS

Federal, state, and local funding, as well as private payment from seniors has resulted in a rich array of programs in many communities. Senior

Centers are a hub for social and educational opportunities. Adult day care centers, both social and medical, have emerged, addressing a variety of needs for their clients while providing respite for the family or an informal support system that cares for the individual when returned to the community. Nursing homes are also being used as a respite location, to allow families to regroup for up to two weeks, allowing for family vacations that might otherwise not be possible. Transportation systems have been developed to allow for seniors to interact within the greater community, preventing episodes of isolation.

Home health care is important. Following a hospital stay this service may be necessary for the older person's recuperation and return to optimal functioning. Personal care workers, attendant care, home health aides, homemaker services, chore services (housekeeping, shopping), companion and respite service, and home-delivered meals are all part of a complex of formal and informal services that are largely taken for granted until one becomes frail, infirm, or sick. The presence of family or informal caregivers along with the formal delivery services maximizes the positive outcome for the senior.

## HOUSING OPTIONS FOR OLDER ADULTS

Developers have addressed senior housing needs through a variety of models. Affordable housing, independent housing, independent housing with services, enriched housing, supportive housing, assisted living, and continuing care retirement communities are some of the types of housing that people may need to investigate as they grow older. The decision is often based on many considerations, including locality (urban, suburban, or rural), health status, income level, assets, and ongoing expected monthly income. Some of these models work well if a senior has social security, pension income, annuity income, or other sources of funds, including support from adult children. Too much income might exclude a senior from moving into a particular type of housing environment, as might too little income for some other options. Public housing or federally supported housing generally serves the low income members of our society, whereas Continuing Care Communities provide upscale housing to seniors with significant means.

### Independent Housing

Independent housing arrangements are living arrangements for seniors living alone or with a spouse who are able to make most decisions about their living activity on a daily basis without the assistance of others. They may live in their own home or apartment or in congregate living arrangement or senior communities. Within this type of housing it is possible for an individual to receive some supportive services.

## Supportive Housing

Supportive housing options usually become necessary when the senior's condition deteriorates or becomes complicated, perhaps due to chronic conditions further restricting personal independence. The variety of supportive housing options has grown rapidly in recent years with differing costs, services, and living arrangements. Although definitions vary by state, four major types of supportive housing can be described.

### Subsidized Housing Programs

Many older persons live in federally subsidized housing for renters with low incomes. According to research conducted by the AARP's public policy institute, roughly 1.7 million older persons live in federally subsidized housing. The Section 202 Elderly Housing Program is the primary federal program to construct subsidized rental housing for older adults. The public housing and section 8 rental assistance programs also serve large numbers of older persons. Many housing facilities have service coordinators on staff who provide supportive services such as group meals, housekeeping, and transportation (Kochera, 2001).

### Board and Care Homes

Board and care homes provide protective oversight, meals, and limited assistance with activities of daily living. According to a 1995 study, as many as one million people may live in board and care homes (Hawes, Mor, & Wildfire, 1995). Many of these homes also service residents with mental retardation, developmental disabilities, and some with mental illness. There are also homes that serve mixed-resident populations including older persons with physical and cognitive disabilities. Adult foster care homes are separately licensed in some states to provide services for two to five residents in a small, homelike environment (Gibson, 2003).

### Assisted Living

Assisted living is a state-regulated and monitored residential long-term care option. It provides or coordinates oversight and services to meet the residents' individualized scheduled needs, based on their assessments and service plans, and their unscheduled needs as they arise.

Services that are required by state law must include but are not limited to:

- 24-hour awake staff to provide oversight and meet scheduled and unscheduled needs
- Provision and oversight of personal and supportive services (assistance with activities of daily living and instrumental activities of daily living)
- Health-related services (e.g., medication management services)
- Social services
- Recreational activities
- Meals
- Housekeeping and laundry
- Transportation

A resident has the right to make choices and receive services in a way that will promote the resident's dignity, autonomy, independence, and quality of life. These services are disclosed and agreed to in the contract between provider and resident. Assisted living does not generally provide ongoing, 24-hour skilled nursing (Assisted Living Workgroup, 2003).

### Continuing Care Retirement Communities (CCRCs)

Continuing are retirement communities, often referred to a "Corks," are usually campus-like settings that include private apartments and/or freestanding homes, assisted living, and skilled nursing services. Approximately 80% of CCRCs are sponsored by nonprofit organizations, and more than two-thirds include substantial up-front fees with guarantees of increasing levels of services as residents' needs change.

Almost all residents pay privately, at least in the independent and assisted living sections. In 2001, nearly 2,200 CCRCs in the United States served approximately 650,000 residents, of whom roughly half (320,000) were in independent apartments, 115,000 were in assisted living units, and 215,000 were in nursing home units (Fitch Ratings, & National Investment Center, 2002).

For those older people who are becoming frail and in need of living assistance, including community-based services, home health care, and social services in general, these services are usually dependent on the individual's having adequate housing. The future older population, as mentioned in chapter 1, will be more educated, have higher income and assets, and therefore expect to have more choices about where they will live. Although the housing options mentioned above have specific requisites, all possibilities should be explored before final decisions are made in order to ensure quality of life until the end of life.

## CONCLUSION

The major problems for elders lie in housing for the poor and others who require assistance. When national resources are limited, it is very tempting to focus attention on more achievable minor housing goals. Despite their value for people with special needs and limited resources, such programs as home equity conversion, the many forms of alternative housing, condominium-conversion protection, pension-fund investment in housing, Section 202, congregate housing, and a family subsidy for caregiving, can only address some but not all of the housing needs.

Scarcity of resources in segments of our society are becoming more apparent. In many instances the gap between the classes is expanding to the elimination of a middle class. The very wealthy generally have means to address their social and health needs into old age; the very poor may be served through a safety net provided by federal, state, and local programs; the middle class may become society's next major public policy concern. Discussion of entitlements and who will fund what particular program will continue. Medicaid has, for most states, become the single largest expenditure for government and therefore, in time of scarcity, has become the main target for reduction, recognizing that most states revenue is tax based. Competition for federal and state funding is expected to intensify.

Future leaders in the long-term care arena will be expected to navigate this complex continuum, re-engineer its organization, redefine its mission, and articulate a strategic vision to carry it forward in meeting the needs of the community at large. It is clear that quality care will be the most necessary value for the long-term care continuum.

## REFERENCES

American Association of Homes and Services for the Aging. (2003, August). *Unpublished policy position papers for federal advocacy*. Washington DC.

Assisted Living Workgroup. (2003, April). *Assisted living*. Final report to the United States Senate Special Committee on Aging.

Bowers, B. J. (2000). The relationship between staffing and quality in long-term care facilities: Exploring the views of nurse aides. *Journal of Nursing Care Quality, 14*(4), 43–46.

Cantor, M. (1979). The informal support system, its relevance in the lives of the elderly. In E. Borgotta & N. McCluskey (Eds.), *Aging and society* (pp. 2–6). Beverly Hills, CA: Sage.

Centers for Medicare & Medicaid Services. (2003, November). *Skilled Nursing Facility, Prospective Payment Systems (SNF PPS)*, available at http://www.cms.hhs.gov/providers/snfpps

Federal Interagency Forum on Aging-Related Statistics. (2000, August). *Older Americans 2000: Key indicators of well-being* (p. 46). Federal Interagency Forum on Aging-Related Statistics, Washington, DC: U.S. Government Printing Office.

Fitch Ratings and National Investment Center. (2002). *Investment analysis of continuing care retirement communities.* Annapolis, MD: National Investment Center.

General Accounting Office. (2001). *Nursing workforce: Recruitment and retention of nurses and nurses aides are a growing concern.* Statement of William Scanlon, Director, Health Care Issues. GAO-01-75OT.

General Accounting Office. (2003, July). *Nursing home quality: Prevalence of serious problems, while declining, reinforces importance of enhanced oversight.* Available at http://www.gao.gov/new.items/d03561.pdf

Gibson, M. J. (2003). Meshing services with housing: Lessons for adult foster care and assisted living in Oregon. *Beyond 50: A report to the nation on independent living and disability* (p. 76). Washington, DC: AARP Public Policy Institute.

Hawes, C., Mor, V., & Wildfire, J. (1995). *Analysis of the effect of regulation on the quality of care in board and care homes* (pp. 12–29). Washington, DC: Department of Health and Human Services.

Kane, R. A. (2003). Definition, measurement, and correlates of quality of life in nursing homes: Toward a reasonable practice, research and policy agenda. *The Gerontologist (23)*2, 28–36.

Kochera, A. (2001). A summary of Federal rental housing programs. *Public policy institute fact sheet #85.* Washington, DC: AARP.

Long, W. R., Street, W., Tannenbaum, F., & Johnson, H. (2003). *Historic asylums.* Available at http://www.rootsweb.com/~asylums/mainpage.html

Manard, B. (2002, December). *Nursing home quality indicators: Their uses and limitations.* Available at http://research.aarp.org/health/inb62homes.pdf

McDonald, C. A. (1994). Recruitment, retention and recognition of frontline workers in long-term care. *Generations, 15*(3), 41–42.

Merliss, M. (1999, September). *Financing long-term care in the twenty-first century: The public and private roles.* Available at The Commonwealth Fund: http://cmwf.org/programs/elders/merlis_longtermcare21st.asp

National Center for Health Statistics. (2002, September). *National nursing home survey.* Available at http://www.cdc.gov/nchs/about/major/nnhsd.htm

Ong, P. M., Rickles, J., Matthias, R., & Benjamin, A. E. (2002). *California caregivers: Final labor market analysis.* Report to the California Employment Development Department.

Pillemer, K., Hegeman, C., Dean, C., Albright, B., & Meador, R. (1997). *Partners in caregiving, cooperative communication between families and nursing homes* (p. 3). Cornell Gerontology Research Institute Report.

Stone, R. I. (2003, October). *Why workforce development should be part of the long-term care quality debate.* Paper prepared by the Institute for the Future of Aging Services.

Stone, R. I., Harahan, M. F., Kiefer, K. M., Johnson, A. B., Guiliano, J., & Bowers, B. (2003, June). Addressing shortages in the direct care workforce: The recruitment and retention practices of California's not-for-profit nursing homes, continuing care retirement communities and assisted living facilities (pp. 28–29). Washington DC: The Institute for the Future of Aging Services.

U.S. Administration on Aging. (2003, October). *Aging Internet information notes on nursing homes.* Available at: http://www.aoa.gov/prof/notes/notes_nursing_homes.asp

U.S. Department of Health and Human Services. (2003, March). *Nursing home deficiency trends and survey and certification process consistency.* Office of Inspector General. Available at http://oig.hhs.gov/oei/reports/oei-02-01-00600.pdf.

# 4

# Environmental Design in Evoking the Capacities of Older People

## Lorraine G. Hiatt

One can barely pick up a professional journal or national newspaper without reading about health care staffing shortages, costs of care, and the likely impact on the existing resources of seven million aging "boomers" (American Association of Homes and Services for the Aging [AAHSA], 1997; Anderson, Hsieh, & Su, 1998; Harrington, O'Meara, Kitchener, Simon, & Schnelle, 2003). What's newsworthy? Perhaps it's a sense of vulnerability. We appear to be caught in a generation that asks for health care, and providers who settle for traditional institutional images and organization (Vladeck, 1980), working from the script of Goffman's *Asylums* (1961). Both sponsors and families may overlook the possibilities for good looking, responsive and effectively operating health care (Wagner & Creelman, 2004; Brunk, 1998).

Wouldn't it be terrific if seniors' environments could play a meaningful role in successful aging? Such a vision could promote greater independence and improve the social context for friends, family, and caregivers (Werezak & Morgan, 2003). Even better, what if environmental design were effective and fiscally feasible and choices were readily available!

The purpose of this chapter is to identify the interplay between health care of seniors and the environment; to outline uses of environment in routines of direct caregiving and indirect ancillary support; and to propose ways these considerations can contribute to a more appropriate "culture" or focus of health care for seniors and for providers of care. The emphasis follows literature available to date, which has more to say about facility-based living environments than it does about households and wellness settings. This chapter may also be read as a professional challenge to use the tools of health care and gerontological training to respond to important questions and address unmet needs.

## EXAMPLES OF CONCERNS FOR ENVIRONMENTAL GERONTOLOGY

1. *Functional Independence:* Can environmental modifications (sensory, functional access) increase independence and capacities for conducting instrumental activities of daily living (Bosman, 1994; Windley & Scheidt, 1980)? How might this apply to people at home? "Smarter" houses (Hiatt, 1988) and technology that connects distant caregivers and seniors are ways of keeping seniors at home, and perhaps in more interesting environments (Gitlin, 2003).

2. *Assisted Independence:* What roles can assisted living play in supporting seniors who seek special residences in response to physical, social, psychological, or temporal needs? (Frytak, Kane, Finch, Kane, & Maude-Griffin, 2001; Zimmerman et al., 2003). How can assistance be afforded without overlooking individual choices and life patterns (Kane, Caplan, Urv-Wong, et al., 1997)? Is "aging in place," remaining in your own housing, a viable concept (Chapin & Dobbs-Kepper, 2001) and what design features facilitate success? What policies are needed to support the development of assisted living in the U.S. (Mollica, 1998)?

3. *Memory and Judgment:* What is possible for memory-impaired persons to achieve in health care (Gwyther, 1997)? What role does the overall environment play in cueing or confusing the behavior of cognitively impaired persons (Cohen & Day, 1993)? What are the person–environment design priorities given various patterns, stages, or capacities in senile dementia, Alzheimer's type dementia, or related disorders (Day, Carreon, & Stump, 2000)? How effective are external, environmental design features in providing information, and on supporting lapses in judgment or abstract reasoning (Sloane, Linderman, Phillips, Morita, & Koch, 1995)?

4. *Healing and Palliative Care:* Environment stimuli are beginning to be respected for seniors who are receiving comfort care in the process of restoration, habilitation, or dying. At one point, only free-standing hospices were more focused on these features. Now, they may be equally applicable in wellness programs and facilities, assisted living, and home environments (Chiazzi, 2000; Hannen, 2003).

5. *Culture of Care and Design:* What is the "culture" of the care environment? How can it be adapted or recrafted to provide a more fulfilling life for those engaged in necessary health care (focus on activities of

daily living such as mobility, agility, endurance, transfer, continence, eating, bathing and skin care, sleeping, dressing, communications, and cognition (Hiatt, 1988)?

6. *Social Experiences, Numbers of People/Roles and Size:* How might size of the social setting, complexity, service goals, and configuration (square footage) figure into the desired outcomes of senior living and care? Can appropriate design reduce boredom and promote social exchange (Boyd, 2003; Werezak & Morgan, 2003)?

7. *Lifelong Development and Design:* Can more thoughtful organization and management of the major personal or living environments contribute to a more positive developmental (vs. compartmentalized) notion of senior health care (a focus on aging despite decline, considering the many categories of dependence) (Golant, 2003; Thomas & Johansson, 2003).

8. *Environmental Decisions and Staffing Levels:* Do environmental design decisions have an impact on scarce staffing? How can the environment support the costly service of "vigilance," including oversight? (Mahoney, 2003).

9. *Quantification of Space, Configuration, and Technology:* How do amount of space, layouts, technologies, organization, and design influence the effectiveness of care, attract and retain labor? How significant are these in particular settings or for seniors with particular constellations of need?

10. *The New Math of Functional Design:* What if seniors experience further decline, "age in place," or require new nursing home beds? How can environmental planning address initial needs and changes or flexibility in demand? How should the components of what people pay for (capital and soft costs, the care itself, and consumables) be quantified into economic models designed toward the results we seek, rather than the systems and facilities inherited from the hospital model of care?

11. *More Informed Environmental Design:* What is the object of more informed environmental design for seniors? The seldom asked question at the crux of design is this: If we were to appropriately design and configure space, providing sufficient area and appropriate technology to the particular time and space needs of the senior, would we reduce more costly and restrictive institutionalization? What benchmarks are needed to incorporate environmental design considerations at various price points and in projects funded by governmental or public resources? For sponsors to commission architects and builders to incorporate improvements in space, layout, technologies and materials, they and the state governments who review plans (and pay through Medicaid reimbursements), will need better data (Dimotta, Dubey, Hoglund, &

Kershner, 1993). Benchmarks may lead to informed choices regarding how particular combinations of design decisions would affect the true daily costs of nursing home care and the actual productive time available for staff in caregiving.

- What are planning and construction related costs for functional room layouts, more individual rooms and bathrooms, for floor plans organized to support workflow of nursing assistants as well as that of nurses, food service staff, and materials management?
- What are the demonstrable outcomes for residents, including those affecting physical health (mobility and balance; falls; skin problems; ability to make needs known; sleep; or, nutrition), emotional and mental well-being (agitation; attention, responsiveness); and the implications of these on costs of care including direct care staffing?
- What is the interaction of design and length of stay, use of hospitals, cost of medications and other treatments? Quantifying any such savings would help rethink the distribution of expenditures, with important implications for governments as well as families paying for care themselves?
- Do better designed buildings help attract and retain staff; reduce job-related stress; reduce physical injury to staff (in lifting, for example)? Such outcomes need to be expressed in terms of human satisfaction (reduced stress; increased satisfaction with resident interactions) as well as their operational costs (Gnaedinger, 2003).
- How do particular design decisions or floor plans impact specific staff time available for the management minutes needed for 1-1 toilet training, improved dining, more effective mobility, and better attention to cognition and memory support? We lack benchmarks on the combined impact of multiple improvements; i.e., those addressing room area and more compact building configurations. To address private rooms without improving walking distances on all three shifts, may be to add inconvenience and staffing time without achieving more familiar, residential scale or image.

## BACKGROUND LITERATURE

### Theoretical Progress in Environmental Gerontology

Environmental gerontology grew from the efforts of ethnographers and environmental social scientists (Bechtel & Churchman, 2002; Walsh,

Craik, & Price, 2000). As of yet, environmental issues are seen as a transaction system: acting upon the person and being acted upon by the person. The environment is not a single, controlled feature with generalized outcomes, despite what popular literature may suggest about wall color producing behavior (Wahl & Weisman, 2003).

M. Powel Lawton, an early theoretical contributor to environmental gerontology, collaborated with a wide number of peers and developed a descriptive theory, as well as empirical research on how environments inadvertently "press" upon behavior, independence, satisfaction, and lifestyles (Lawton & Nahemow, 1973).

Environment, by nature, engages a broad domain of topics. Controlled environmental and behavioral research has not met academic requirements for elegant theory and clean scientific research. Wahl and Weisman (2003) have attempted to analyze the empirical environmental gerontology literature published from 1989 to 2000, admittedly focusing on *PsychInfo* sources. By their count, the body of empirical studies numbers fewer than 50 articles a year. Day, Carreon, and Stump (2000) have made a similar effort to analyze findings in dementia outcomes, many of which have addressed issues of environment, with varying results. The state of research needs to challenge the bravura of good generalists in aging who enter into actual design decisions. Lack of sound research suggests the need to sift findings, to speak in terms of "indicators," and to reject single cause–effect design–behavior imperatives (Wylde, 1997). Excellent commentaries on theoretical advances were written by Golant (2003), Wahl and Weisman (2003), and Gitlin (2003). There is no firm foundation, nor is there any sound research supporting suggestions that a color "produces" behavior, relaxing or otherwise (Tofle, Schwarz, & Max-Royale, 2004). As another pioneer in environmental gerontology noted, "environments are as hypotheses in human aging research" (Howell, 1980).

Golant (2003) captures a strategic vision for future environmental studies:

> It is not just the safety or friendliness of an environment that is most valued, but rather the regular and predictable morning walk in the neighborhood; it is not just the presence of grab bars in the bathroom that is important, but the ability and confidence to shower safely; it is not a friendship that is supportive of expressive or instrumental needs, but the regular twice-weekly visit with a friend; and it is not just the staff–resident ratio that is significant to the residents in an assisted living facility, but rather the timeliness of staff–resident transactions and whether residents' specific personal needs are met as a result of staff actions. [pp. 643–644]

Where does this leave professionals managing or working in health care and assisted living environments? The reality is the tendency for "others" to create the environment; then the managing professionals figure out how it should be staffed, lacking valuable input from "participatory design" as well as insight from peer-reviewed projects (American Institute of Architects, 2002).

After consulting to, researching, and visiting over 800 U.S. facilities of many types, the author has observed that the lack of a system for incorporating available information into design has led to costly facilities that fragment services, frustrate staff, and alienate if not immobilize seniors. This disconnection among direct care, ancillary support services, and dwelling design unnecessarily burdens both seniors and caregivers.

## DESIGN IMPLICATIONS FOR SENIORS WITH IMPLICATIONS FOR THEIR CAREGIVERS

For professionals to adequately evaluate, communicate with, or negotiate with seniors, it is often helpful to consider the impact of context on the experience of a situation. Germain (1977) has even advanced the concept of an "ecologically valid environment" for some psychosocial and related functional assessments. What considerations might be addressed by professionals who are not in a position to construct environments, but might select or shape situations to advantage? Environments communicate images and expectations; there is a potential for the setting to evoke images of capability or images supporting ennui and idleness or even learned helplessness (Marsden, 2001). Therefore, environments contribute to feelings that may carry over to an interview or evaluation setting.

## MARKETING RETIREMENT HOUSING

Marketing retirement housing and health care has been one application of this line of study. Seniors are increasingly clear proponents of environmental design. Fox, Schur, and Ejaz (2003) reported that a third of the negative comments of retirement community seniors addressed physical design features. This represented the highest of any category of criticisms.

Positive images for environments and products have received new attention since the late 1980s, prompted by the desire to distinguish retirement housing and assisted living from health care (Goodman &

Smith, 1992) and to market products for independence that looked so good they did not draw attention to possible frailities (Selvidge, Wylde, & Rummage, 1993). What image is "senior friendly" or "non-institutional?" Responses typically show geographic variations and distinctions based on one's present need or "timing" (Gitlin, 2003; Golant, 2003). Ethnographic input from seniors themselves, who are satisfied with their sense of familiar, of home, would be valuable in teasing out significant priorities. The topic or domain of "home" seems to produce more descriptive imagery, especially for some physically limited and memory-impaired persons (Baldwin, 2002).

Marsden's studies (2001) have operationalized the essence of a home as it should be applied to an actual house, enclosure, human scale (small and familiar) and natural features. Such findings support the emergence of building floor plans for nursing care, assisted living, and dementia care that reduce emphasis on corridors and tinker with room arrangements to create neighborhoods, clusters of care, small group living, and ways of reducing the scale and institutional impact of traditional health care environments (Hiatt, 1991a, 1991c; Mikelson & Johnson, 2003; Thomas & Johansson, 2003). Critics of health care environments protest its unfamiliar qualities, seeking to find a more familiar home-like environment.

## Compensation

Features of the environment may instrumentally compensate for diminished sensory function. Improvements in lighting levels and reductions in glare, for example, appear to improve contrast visibility for some seniors (Bosman, 1994; Brawley & Taylor, 2001). There may be a role for full-spectrum or natural light in senior environments (Mishima, Okawa, Hozumi, & Hishikawa, 2000). Modifications of visual and acoustical settings seem to improve concentration and may have a positive effect on access of the "memory vault" (Fozard, 1981; Voeks, Gallagher, Langer, & Drinka, 1990). Other features may have a palliative effect (making one feel better about the walk rather than actually producing mobility). Shorter walking distances may help one feel more energetic and mobile (Ferrell, 2000); reduced background noise may contribute to lessened sense of confusion and/or agitation (Hogland & Ledewitz, 1999).

## Memory Support

Environmental design features, objects including external stimuli such as music or pets, may cue or evoke recall or stimulate appropriate responses. Environmental design may also be valuable in reducing reliance on abstract reasoning. Higher order intelligence is often flawed through multi-infarct dementia or senile dementia of the Alzheimer's type (Fozard, 1981). Environmental design features may also support activities of daily living for memory-impaired persons, perhaps playing a role in continence management (Briller, Proffitt, Perez, Calkins, & Marsden, 2001) and general "independence" (Namazi & Johnson, 2002).

## Environmental Detractors and Barriers to Communications

Ill-suited or poorly managed environmental features may mitigate attention, and impede the effectiveness of learning or sensory processing (Hiatt, 1987b). Background noise, traffic, lack of fresh air, overly or under-stimulating surroundings may all blunt the capacity for thinking (Bosman, 1994).

## Mobility, Agility and Endurance

The arrangement of the physical environment, of entries, fixtures, and features, may facilitate movement, safe transfer of weight, balance, success in bearing weight, and the breadth of one's social contacts (Bourrett, Bernick, Cott, & Kontos, 2002; Hiatt, 1988; Hoenig, Pieper, Zolkewitz, Schenkman, & Branch, 2002). Maintaining mobility appears to be a possible method of sustaining seniors in more independent environments (Kiely, Leveille, & Morris, 2002). Improved seating may maximize comfort and ease of standing (Hiatt, 1991c).

## ENVIRONMENTAL DESIGN AND ALZHEIMER'S AND RELATED DISORDERS

There are a spate of practitioners who have drawn attention to design methods for dealing with wandering risk in people with dementia (Hoglund & Ledewitz, 1999) and redirecting behavior (Perez, Profit, & Calkins, 2001). Many solutions may work for one individual (who may stop at an exit "stop" sign) but be of little use to others (perhaps because they observe so many going through it). In part, this may be due to a lack of professional understanding of the ravages to abstract reasoning that occur with some forms of dementia coupled with an ardent desire to mitigate wandering risks (Hiatt, 1992).

Abstract reasoning touches on many environmental themes: color coding as a way-finding cue, selecting clothes for today's weather or for an occasion, recalling what one ordered a day before, recalling what procedure or device is needed to summon help. Making and keeping appointments can be particularly vexing. As of this writing, there has been little success in retraining abstract reasoning skills, including safe driving in persons with these deficits.

A follow-up on the topic of color is in order. Combinations of colored objects (contrasting with the forms and tones of the background environment, perhaps), movement, and serendipitous objects have been used to diffuse anxiety in some and elicit attention in others. One system of combining such stimuli in a multisensory room and program is called "snoezelen" and appears useful for profoundly impaired and/ or the most cognitively regressed clients (Kinkead, 2003). The Dutch term "snoezelen," combines words for sniffing (smelling) and snoozing.

## Memory Support and Montessori Approaches to Dementia Care

Memory support is a systematic practice of focusing attention, reducing reliance of flawed reasoning skills, using familiar, simply presented stimuli and supporting the acceptable responses (Hiatt, 1991b; Hiatt, Brandon, & Dunlop, 2001). When the physical and social environment is designed to focus on features that can be used, manipulated and touched and where the goal is to evoke motion and response, without over or under stimulation, this is referred to as a "Montessori approach to memory support" (Hiatt, 1989a). In practice, success in Montessori approaches results from providing eclectic objects and encouraging freedom of movement and "discovery" of interests (Hiatt, 1987b; Camp & Camp, 2001). Individuals may explore individually or be encouraged to small groups. Success is limited when the objects become "cute" untouchable, historically contrived or when features become mere décor and are not connected with meaningful daily life (Hiatt, 1991b; Hiatt, Brandon, & Dunlop, 2001).

The following examples illustrate the combined impact of memory support programs and activities that incorporate architectural changes:

1. *Reduce Noxious Stimuli.* Noise, acrid smells, clutter, and confusing traffic patterns may all reduce attention span and add to agitation, confounding the use of residual memory. These are virtually noxious

stimuli. The adept person can often move away from these stimuli with loss of the capacity to plan; the memory-impaired individual may be more likely to dwell amid stimulus overload. Typically, one manages or redesigns around these factors before implementing environmental interventions (Hiatt, 1991b).

2. *Provide Familiar Stimuli.* Familiar stimuli and objects may offer substance for interventions, especially if incorporated into the design (Olsen, Hutchings, & Ehrenkrantz, 2000). Fresh food aromas may evoke natural digestive juices, stimulating appetite and facilitating the ingestion of food in severely cognitively impaired persons (Carter & Hallett, 2002). Recognizable objects, coupled with practice and verbal reinforcement may aid some in finding target spaces, such as their room in a care facility (Nolan, Mathews, & Harrison, 2001). Fresh air may also contribute to general well-being (Hiatt, 1991a, 1991b, 1991c). Familiar encounters with natural stimuli and people who seem familiar also appear to reduce agitation (Marcus & Barnes, 1999; Whall, Black, Groh, Yankou, Kupferschmidt, & Foster, 1997).

3. *Encourage Full Body Movement.* Use music and exercise to meaningfully occupy time and reduce agitation (Hiatt, 1991a, 1991c; Hiatt, Brandon, & Dunlap, 2001; Remington, 2002). Architecture for people with reduced memory was formerly designed to minimize movement and risk; newer thinking is to encourage freedom of movement in safe and interesting (but secure) surroundings both inside and outside, weather permitting (Hiatt, 1991c; Hoglund & Ledewitz, 1999).

4. *Establish Meaningful Use of Time, Alternatives to Boredom and Sitting.* The quintessential negative image of a traditional nursing home is either lines of people in the hall around a tight central nurses station or halls cluttered with equipment. Assisted living has typically been free of these images (though concerns have been raised about hanging around in lobbies).

Environments need spaces for gathering and tables for putting out things to do (Hiatt, 1987a, 1991c). Staff tasks are sometimes recrafted and/or staff is trained to interact more directly with residents, sometimes referring to objects of personalization or other memorabilia collected by families to stimulate conversation (Altus, Engelman, & Mathews, 2002; Hiatt, 1991c; Kehoe & Van Heesch, in press; Pillemer, 1996; Stone, 2003).

Exceptional staff is often described in terms of capacity to make time for residents (Johnson, 1996). It is not necessary that seniors glean the full impact of the physical cues or conversation for it to be beneficial (Hiatt et al., 2001).

5. *Use Options for Quiet or Calming Settings to Reduce Agitation.* Environmental design, ranging from group size and noise to provision of objects and vulnerability to destruction or risk, may all have roles in egging on or reducing disruptive behaviors (Hiatt, 1989; Souder & O'Sullivan, 2003). This option may include privacy or private territory within a shared space (Hiatt, 1991c; Marsden, 2001).

6. *Have a Curriculum or Concept: Blend Concept and Design Priorities.* Merely providing a secure or distinct space or unit appears to have little impact on slowing cognitive decline (Philips et al., 1997). Positive outcomes in use of the setting may relate to how one lives rather than whether abstract reasoning and judgment return (Hiatt et al., 2001).

## ENVIRONMENTAL DESIGN AND TRANSFORMATION OF NURSING HOMES: THE LANGUAGE OF "CULTURE CHANGE"

Late in the 1990s there emerged a series of factors that have influenced thinking about outcomes for seniors who undergo changes affecting activities of daily living, instrumental activities of daily living, physical functioning, cognition, judgment, and responses to life itself. Increasingly, these are referred to as a "culture change." Themes of those engaged in redefining the culture of caring environments have direct implications for environmental design planning. The following are some highlights of culture change themes in care facilities:

1. Client-focused schedules (Gnaedinger, 2003), and self-directed health care (Stone, 2003)
2. Reduced social scale (small groups of 6–12 rather than 20–60 for meals) (Boyd, 2003)
3. Meaningful use of time (Boyd, 2003; Brennan, Branaccio, & Brecanier, 2003)
4. Increased natural qualities of environments (MacKenzie, 2003)
5. Familiarization of routines of care including dining with choices in familiar settings and with fresh aromas (Brennan, Brancaccio, & Brecanier, 2003); bathing improvements (Sloane, 2001), and more familiar night experiences (Mather, Nemecek, & Oliver, 1997)
6. Improved social encounters in naturally collaborative activities stressed over one-sided caregiving (Thomas & Johansson, 2003) and time viewed as precious (Boyd, 2003).

## The Eden Alternative: A Case Study of Environmental Change

The work of Thomas and Johansson (Thomas & Johannson, 2003) and Fagan (2003) has led to a major grass-roots effort to change the culture of nursing homes. Thomas's initial efforts to naturalize the environment through the Eden movement have had far-reaching effects, most recently in providing detached small "Green Houses™." "The Eden Alternative designs an environment that has all the requisite medication and treatment facilities but does not make them the axis around which the elder's world turns. We're making the axis the plants, the pets, the children, the relationships, and the garden" (Thomas & Johansson, 2003, p. 284).

## Outcome Data of Culture Change

Although the outcome data are relatively new (and short-term), findings have addressed the significance of new lifestyles and family participation, new roles for staff (Mahoney, 2003; Wilkerson & MacDonald, 2003), and implications for policy (Harrington, Zimmerman, Karon, Robinson, & Buetel, 2000). No single organization or set of organizations holds itself as the prototype service, size, or model of desired outcomes; this harks to the fact that differences in concept, programs, price point, and location will stimulate demand for a variety of choices in later life experiences.

There are examples from for-profit settings (Hagy, 2003), state and veterans facilities (Valentine, 1998), and numerous examples from non-profit organizations (Brennan et al., 2003). Critics often wonder whether culture change is real or the newest label to distinguish a "boutique" senior service. Those listed in the case examples are engaged in more than superficial program distinction. However, it is fair to ask what implementing a deeper range of initiatives will mean to the 17,000 existing licensed nursing care facilities (Bond & Fiedler, 1999; Rosenfield & Wyatt, 1984), though that has not stopped some pioneers from abandoning traditional large nursing homes with their long corridors, institution-driven schedule, and departmental structure from developing smaller, resident-centered "houses" (Mikelson & Johnson, 2003; Gnaediger, 2003).

Some question whether small scale experiences and diversified staffing roles can be achieved in dense, urban settings with high real estate costs. The groundswell grass-roots innovation (Fagan, 2003; SAGE, 2003) as well as research suggests that organizations with a cultural alternative to more institutional nursing homes or assisted living residences will become a market choice (Stone, 2003).

## THE SIGNIFICANCE OF ENVIRONMENTAL DESIGN TO DIRECT CAREGIVERS

The national shortages of direct caregivers, homecare, assisted living and nursing homes are well documented (Gregory, 2001). According to the National Nursing Home Survey, seventeen thousand licensed nursing homes house nearly 1.5 million residents ages 65 and over (Gabriel, 2000). These facilities are staffed by 1.4 million people, of which 950,000+ are nursing staff, including two-thirds or 617,000 who are Certified Nursing Assistants (CNAs).

Unfortunately, these national staffing analyses and projections are made without reference to building features and design (Health Care Finance Agency, 2000; Wylde, 1997): the facility size and gross area, floor plan, attributes, or configurations. Without such data, it is hard to interpret findings: Three hours of one-on-one care a day may have one implication for a "cluster" designed or small scale environment with conveniently located utilities, gathering areas and a design that flows from the day's routines. However, in a building with lengthy corridors, central facilities, and off-unit social programs, more of that three hours is allocated to searching, walking, and waiting than to individual care. Sadly, a facility may well offer the highest of industry staffing ratios, but that does not mean that the seniors are receiving significant proportional value from these precious resource people.

Environmental design can transform the workplace, the burdensome qualities of care of seniors, and the use of time. There are possibilities both in new construction and in modest renovation of vintage buildings (Boyd, 2003; Hiatt, 1991c). Gnaedinger (2003) has reflected upon the challenges facing culture change organizations and cites, "workload, resistance to change at all levels, 'operational realities,' resident characteristics and the design and scale of the built environment (p. 356). Robyn Stone, with great perspective from the many Wisconsin area Wellspring Projects (projects involving culture change in a group of midwestern nursing homes, funded by The Commonwealth Fund), summarizes similar barriers to culture change, placing additional emphasis on the characteristics of the residential environment and staffing shortages (Stone, 2003; Kehoe & Van Heesch, in press). It is as though caregivers (and to some degree administrators) are spinning off precious time to address limitations in the facilities, deflecting energy from priorities involving contact with residents needing their attention, all because of fear that addressing environmental design will be too costly or is superfluous.

## Recasting the Roles of Staff and Image of Operations

A single national inventory of innovations in service concept, staffing, and design has yet to be assembled. Topics to be addressed in future research and practice need to include the following.

### What Is Direct Caregiving?

What tasks and interchanges need to be considered for people of a particular "case mix" or care profile in a typical shift for a particular point in time? What supportive efforts are also required and also "done" (from communications and charting to being educated)? What nonproductive tasks are fulfilled and can any of these "labor hogs" be mitigated through products and design? Examples might be redesign of centralized laundry, central staff stations, and fixed communications or call systems.

### What Time Is and Could Be Available

It is reported that 3.2–3.4 hours per person per day is a typical standard for nursing care staffing (Harrington, Kovner, Mezey, et al., 2000). From American Association of Retired Persons website data (AARP, 2004), one learns that this translates to an average of 38 nursing assistants (in a 24-hour day) to each 100 residents. One can read a flurry of federal literature suggesting 4.2 hours of nursing care (including administrative, "director of nursing") per person per day (U.S. Centers for Medicare and Medicaid Services, 2001) or the Small Green House™ touting 6.0 hours per day (Thomas & Johansson, 2003). Green House projects, however, tend to use diversified workers; one role includes more than nursing assistant. Despite the need for focused supervision for people with particular behavior and physical needs, there are estimates that some people with memory impairment are spending from three to five hours of their time (wakeful hours in assisted and nursing care) alone (Reed, Lach, Smith, & Birge, 1990). This author is not convinced we really do know how much time is and could be available in licensed nursing care.

To simplify and apply the preceding national data to a single center for care, one might find working in actual people, hours and tasks is more useful because one can translate these proportions into a geometry that begins to achieve design that matches night time (the fewest caregivers) while working equally well during the day.

Issues of staffing in assisted living are similarly complicated by varying definitions of admissions, care possible, design features, amount of staffing, and staff training (Mollica, 1998). Stretching staff assignments and multitasking have been attempted (Guylas, 1998). Sometimes new roles for staff are referred to as creation of "universal workers" (AAHSA, 1997b). It has been this author's experience that the features and design of environments also play a role in the success of these new duty definitions. In more "institutional" environments, diversified duties often engage one in more onerous cleaning tasks. When the food, laundry, distances, and supplies are dealt with in an open plan design, role diversification (with its requisite staff training and mentorship) is more likely to succeed.

## DESIGN MODIFICATIONS AND REDIRECTION OF STAFF TIME

Many who resist change in long-term care fear the costs, presuming that redirecting staff time to residents will add complexity to work flow and labor to the payroll. In general, the problem comes when attempting to increase resident-staff contact time using floor plans adopted from acute care; plans that isolating staff; add steps; centrally locate utilities near nurses rather than near residents and care assistants; scrimp on room and bathroom circulation space and increase immobility or dependency of residents. When we finally have sufficiently responsive floor plans available to create a meaningful research sample, we can begin to look specifically at re-designing work flow and its effects on staff time, to measure how wages are expended across all positions (nursing, laundry, food, housekeeping, administration and allied health) in terms of actually quantifying the price for successful completion of tasks, meaningful interactions with residents (for communication, agitation reduction, bathroom and hygiene interventions, appropriate social dining; gait, mobility and balance development; memory enhancement; getting fresh air and even responding to the residents' body rhythms). When we embrace appropriate outcomes and work from effective floor plans, products and technology, we shall be in a better position to model equitable allocation of the total capital and operational costs per person, according to the specific acuities and responses envisioned in re-designed cultures of care.

## A CASE IN POINT: INCONTINENCE, CONTINENCE MANAGEMENT, STAFFING, AND DESIGN

One of the major factors for both families and assisted living providers in placing a senior in a nursing care setting is incontinence management (Hope, Keene, Gedling, Fairburn, & Jacoby, 1998). Incontinence is a difficult issue for nursing care (Frantz, Xakellis, Harvey, & Lewis, 2003). From the senior's point of view, issues range from embarrassment in seeking help, receiving help, and shame in leakage affecting socializing. For caregivers, continence management opens the nursing assistant or family member to risks in lifting, transfer, and environmental precautions, and focuses time on one of the least pleasant aspects of caregiving.

Clinical research has suggested the value of combinations of evaluation, scheduled bath, rooming, and in some cases, medication or treatment. Studies of these interventions have been disappointing: in one example, staff simply was not getting residents to the bathroom; several others relate problems to staffing assignments, duties, and levels (shortages) (Ouslander, Maloney, Grasela, Rogers, & Walawander, 2001). However, few intervention protocols, systems, or cost analyses address basic issues of design that may help both seniors and staff in conjunction with other interventions:

1.  Bathrooms designed to meet the Americans with Disability Act do not address the ergonomic issues of seniors (Hiatt, 1988). Typical space requirements for bathrooms in senior living and health care are based upon the 5' turning radius (Goldsmith, 1998) and do not address the actual turning patterns of seniors or floor area used in assisted transfer or lifts (Hiatt, 1991c, illustrated pp. 73–74). The grab bar configuration and seating height recommended in ADA do not appear consistent with the toileting needs and seating/support preferences and behaviors of seniors. This suggests that in meeting minimum codes, bathroom design for purpose-built senior housing and health care is not meeting seniors' needs (Sanford & Megrew, 1995), making seniors less independent (Hiatt, 1991c).
2.  Bathrooms are typically not designed for safe transfer, which involves consideration of multiple methods of mobility, devices, and assistance patterns.

3. Entries are typically too narrow and door design typically does not suit either independent or assisted toileting, adding time to the process (time that is not easily managed by seniors and time that takes from other seniors).
4. The number of bathrooms is often poorly matched to the needs of seniors. Many times, bathrooms are not available within steps of the mobility-impaired senior (a consideration in conventional housing, as well as assisted living and nursing care).
5. Several labor studies indicate that frequency of toileting assistance is not sufficient to improve continence (Schnelle, Cadogan, Yoshii, et al., 2003) and as a result, both continent and incontinent residents may be receiving similarly low average assists, estimated as an unacceptable 1.3 per day (Schnelle, Cadogan, Grbic, et al., 2003).

Improvement of the design features noted above might increase self-toileting and reduce the use of some transfer lifts (used when a wheelchair will not fit in the bathroom or through the door or when staff cannot get by the wheelchair to close the door). Improved design could further reduce the number of two-person transfers. There is every evidence to suggest that improved bathroom design, overall, may also reduce caregiver back injuries, another source of operational cost (disability pay, insurance, litigation). If we could only get seniors and their caregivers *out* of the bathroom (and free of emotional concerns with toileting), there might be time to provide the vigilance and oversight for behaviors such as wandering or agitation that characterize some people with dementias (Reed et al., 1990).

## Finding More Time for Direct Care: Other Issues

Similar findings on staff shortages have been reported for dining (Kayser-Jones & Schell, 1997; Pearson, Fitzgerald, & Nay, 2003) and dehydration (Kayser-Jones, Sobell, Porter, Barbaccia, & Shaw, 1998). Arguments can be made that in addition to the objectives of those services, there is a role for more efficient space and feature design to extend the effectiveness of staff. Yet another intriguing topic is the health and cost implications of offering private rooms. Two facilities have reported that one person can care for more older people when those residents are in private rooms with private bathrooms (in both cases, the corridors were shortened by "clustering"). The Harry and Jeanette Weinberg campus in Getzville, New York, a peer recognized retirement community and Peter Drucker Award winner, reported fewer infections when residents were cared for in private rooms with toilets vs. shared occupancy rooms and shared bathrooms. Neither report is definitive. However, it would be useful to be able to analyze the labor and capital implications of such features, especially those that become the basic building blocks of design.

## MATH, BENCHMARKS, AND KEYS TO UNLEASHING THE POTENTIAL OF ENVIRONMENTAL DESIGN

Proportionately, capital costs, those expenditures related to facilities, furnishings, equipment, and related professional costs (including financing), account for 8% of each person's daily charges (Health Care Information Association [HCIA] & Arthur Anderson, 2000); 15% is allocated to "indirect costs" (maintenance, housekeeping, and food). Of the remaining 62%, 36.5% is allocated to direct care (nursing, social services, activity, and ancillary) and 26% is described as administrative costs. The remaining amount goes to many other things. Too often, policy and boardroom discussions focus on capital costs and labor shortages, without connecting the options for addressing direct and perhaps administrative costs through design. In 2000, $92 billion was collected in nursing home revenues of which 61% was paid for by governmental sources (taxes) (HCIA & Arthur Anderson, 2000). Any other industry spending that kind of money would want product (facility) as well as operations research!

One construct of the culture change projects and their emphasis on smaller environments is to redirect decisions and resources from administration to direct care (Thomas & Johansson, 2003). Would design analysis suggest that labor intensive services in one area could be mitigated through design, allowing different staff assignments for the same bottom line? For example, by reducing labor-intensive floor polishing, might hours (and dollars) be shifted to home-style dining assistance?

True benchmarks of cost of care per person per day and the proportion contributed by capital, operations, and consumables against design features will provide some of the math necessary to realize new approaches to care by design. This is likely to be a challenge to a team of thoughtful, well-trained professionals. When the math and spread sheet analyses are applied to the right questions, we will likely find ways to direct those dollars to a lifestyle of our liking!

## REFERENCES

Altus, D. E., Engelman, K. K., & Mathews, R. M. (2002). Finding a practical method to increase engagement of residents on a dementia care unit. *American Journal of Alzheimer's Disease and Other Dementias, 17*(4), 245–248.

American Association of Homes and Services for the Aging. (1997a). *Summary of assisted living licensure statues and regulations in the 50 states and scope of care.* Washington, DC: Author. Also available at: http//:www/aahsa.org

American Association of Homes and Services for the Aging. (1997b). *The universal worker: Cross-training for organizational change.* Washington, DC: Author.

American Association of Retired Persons. (2004). *The nursing home workforce: Certified nursing assistants.* Available at http://research.aarp.org/health/fs86_cna.html

American Institute of Architects. (2000). *Design for aging review.* Washington, DC: AIA Bookstore and Gloucester, MA: Rockport. Also available at: www.AIA. org.

American Institute of Architects. (2002). *Guidelines for design and construction of hospital and health care facilities 2001.* Washington, DC: Author.

Anderson, R. A., Hsieh, P., & Su, H. (1998). Resource allocation and resident outcomes in nursing homes: Comparisons between the best and worst. *Research in Nursing and American Journal of Azlheimer's Disease Health, 21*, 297–313.

Baldwin, D. (2002, January 10). Main Street as Memory Lane. *New York Times, House and Home* pp. F1, F7.

Bechtel, R., & Churchman, A. (2002). *Handbook of environmental psychology.* New York: Wiley.

Bond, G. E., & Fiedler, F. E. (1999). Culture change: A comparison of leadership vs. renovation in changing staff values. *Nursing Economics, 17*(1), 37–43.

Bosman, C. N. (1994). Age-related changes in perceptual and psychomotor performance: Implications for engineering design. *Experimental Aging Research, 20*(1), 45–59.

Bourrett, E. M., Bernick, L. G., Cott, C. A., & Kontos, P. C. (2002). The meaning of mobility for residents and staff in long-term care facilities. *Journal of Advanced Nursing, 37*(4), 338–345.

Boyd, C. K. (2003). The Providence Mount St. Vincent experience. *Journal of Social Work in Long Term Care, 2*(1), 245–268.

Brancaccio, P., Brecanier, P., & Brennan, J. S. (2004). Teresian House: Using the environment to support culture change. *Journal of Social Work in Long Term Care, 2*(3/4). See Haworthpress.com

Brawley, E., & Taylor, M. (2001). Strategies for upgrading senior care environments: Designing for vision. *Nursing Homes, 50*(6), 28–30.

Brennan, J. S., Brancaccio, P., & Brecanier, P. (2003). Teresian House: Using the environment to support cultural change. *Journal of Social Work in Long Term Care, 2*(1), 223–231.

Briller, S., Proffit, M. A., Perez, K., Calkins, M. P., & Marsden, J. P. (2001). Maximizing cognitive and functional abilities. *Creating successful dementia care settings.* Baltimore: Health Facilities Press.

Brunk, D. (1998). Why people hate long-term care. What's behind the industry's bad public image and what can providers do to improve it? *Contemporary Longterm Care, 21*(1), 38–40.

Burgio, L. D., Allen-Burge, R., Roth, D. L., Bourgeois, M. S., Dijkstra, K., Gerstile, J., Jackson, E., & Bankester, L. (2001). Come talk with me: Improving communication between nursing assistants and nursing home resident during care routines. *The Gerontologist, 41*(4), 449–460.

Camp, C., & Camp, C. J. (2001). *Montessori based activities for persons with dementia.* Baltimore: Health Professionals Press.

Chapin, R., & Dobbs-Kepper, D. (2001). Aging in place in assisted living: Philosophy versus policy. *The Gerontologist, 41*(1), 43–50.

Chiazzi, S. (2000). *The healing home: Creating the perfect place to live with colour, aroma, light and other natural elements.* New York: Trafalgar Square.

Cohen, U., & Day, K. (1993). *Contemporary environments for people with dementia.* Baltimore: Johns Hopkins University Press.

Day, K., Carreon, D., & Stump, C. (2000). Therapeutic design of environments for people with dementia: A review of the empirical research. *Gerontologist, 40*(3), 397–421.

Dimotta, S., Dubey, B. M., Hoglund, D., & Kershner, C. (1993). Long-term care design: Blazing new territory—code reform and beyond. *Journal of Health Care Design, 5,* 197–203.

Fagan, R. M. (2003). *Meeting of pioneers in nursing home culture change. Lifespan: Rochester, NY.* Also available at 716-454-3224, ext 115.

Ferrell, L. S. (2000). Fatigue in an older population. *Journal of the American Geriatric Society, 48*(4), 426–430.

Fox, K., Schur, F., & Ejaz, F. (2003). Residents speak up: Consumer satisfaction in CCRC's. *The Gerontologist, 43,* Special Issue 1, 53. Presentation made at Annual Scientific Meeting, October 5–6.

Fozard, J. L. (1981). Person–environment relationships in adulthood: Implications for human factors engineering. *Human Factors, 23*(1), 7–27.

Frantz, R. A., Xakellis, G. C., Harvey, P. C., & Lewis, A. R. (2003). Implementing an incontinence management protocol in long-term care: Clinical outcomes and cost. *Journal of Gerontological Nursing, 29*(8), 46–53.

Frytak, J. R., Kane, R., Finch, M. D., Kane, R. L., & Maude-Griffin, R. (2001). Outcome trajectories for assisted living and nursing facility residents in Oregon. *Health Services Research, 36,* 91–111.

Gabriel, C. S. (2000). An overview of nursing home facilities: Data from the 1997 National Nursing Home Survey. *Advanced Data Number 311.* Washington, DC: National Center for Health Statistics.

Germain, C. (1977). An ecological perspective on social work practice in health care. *Social Work in Health Care, 3*(1), 67–76.

Gitlin, L. N. (2003). Conducting research on home environments: Lessons learned and new directions. *Gerontologist, 43*(5), 628–637.

Gnaedinger, N. (2003). Changes in long-term care for elderly people with dementia: A report from the front line in British Columbia, Canada. *Journal of Social Work in Long Term Care, 2*(1), 355–371.

Goffman, A. (1961). *Asylums: Essays on the social situation of mental patients and other inmates.* New York: Anchor.

Golant, S. M. (2003). Conceptualizing time and behavior in environmental gerontology: A pair of old issues deserving new thought. *Gerontologist, 43*(5), 638–648.

Goldsmith, S. (1997). *Designing for the disabled: The new paradigm.* New York: Elsevier.

Goodman, R. J., & Smith, D. G. (1992). *Retirement facilities: Planning, design and marketing.* New York: Whitney, Restaurant/Hotel Design International.

Gregory, S. R. (2001). *The nursing home workforce: Certified nurse assistants.* Washington, DC: AARP Public Policy Institute. Also available at AARP.org

Gulyas, R. A. (Ed.). (1998). *The universal worker: Cross-training for organizational change.* Washington, DC: American Association of Homes and Services for the Aging.

Gwyther, L. (1997). The perspectives of persons with Alzheimer's Disease: Which outcomes matter in early and middle stage dementia. *Alzheimer's Disease and Associated Disorders, 11*(6), 18–24.

Hagy, A. (2003). Apple Health Care: Culture change in a privately owned nursing home chain. *Journal of Social Work in Long Term Care, 2*(1), 295–299.

Hannen, S. (2003). *Healing by design.* Lake Mary, FL: Siloam.

Harrington, C., Kovner, C., Mezey, M., Kayser-Jones, J., Burger, S., Mohler, M., Burke, P., & Zimmerman, D. (2000). Experts recommend minimum nurse staffing standards for nursing facilities in the United States. *Gerontologist, 40,* 5–16.

Harrington, C., O'Meara, J., Kitchener, M., Simon, L. P., & Schnelle, J. F. (2003). Designing a report card for nursing facilities: What information is needed and why. *Gerontologist, 43,* Special Issue 11, 47–57.

Harrington, C., Zimmerman, D., Karon, S. L., Robinson, J., & Buetel, P. (2000). Nursing home staffing and its relationship to deficiencies. *Journal of Gerontology, 55*(5), S278–S287.

Health Care Information Association (HCIA) & Arthur Anderson. (2000). *The guide to the nursing home industry 2000.* Baltimore: HCIA, Inc. & Arthur Anderson & Co.

Health Care Finance Agency (HCFA). (2000). *Report to Congress: Appropriateness of minimum nurse staffing ratios in nursing homes.*

Hiatt, L. G. (1982) The environment as a participant in health care. *Journal of Long-Term Care Administration, 10*(1), 1–17.

Hiatt, L. G. (1983). The significance of environmental design to personalized care of older people. In C. Nicholson & J. Nicholson (Eds.), *The personalized care model for the elderly* (pp. 59–89). New York: Department of Mental Hygiene.

Hiatt, L. G. (1987a). The environment's role in the total well-being of the older person. In *Well-being and the elderly: An holistic view* (pp. 23–38). Washington, DC: American Association of Homes for the Aging.

Hiatt, L. G. (1987b). Supportive design for people with memory impairments. In A. Kalicki (Ed.), *Confronting Alzheimer's disease* (pp. 138–164). Owings Mills, MD: National Health Publishing/American Association of Homes for the Aging.

Hiatt, L. G. (1988). Mobility and independence in long-term care: Implications for technology and environmental design. In G. Lesnoff-Caravaglia (Ed.), *Aging in a technological society* (pp. 58–64). New York: Human Sciences Press.

Hiatt, L. G. (1989a). Design and the mentally impaired person: Considerations for the sophisticated sponsor. *Alzheimer's disease: Problems, prospects and perspectives. Vol II* (pp. 393–400). New York: Plenum.

Hiatt, L. G. (1989b). Mental impairment and older people at home. In N. Mace (Ed.), *Dementia care* (pp. 231–242). Baltimore: Johns Hopkins University Press.

Hiatt, L. G. (1991a). Breakthroughs in long term care design. *Journal of Health Care Interior Design, 3,* 205–215.

Hiatt, L. G. (1991b). Designing specialized environments for older people with dementia. In P. Sloan & L. Mattew (Eds.), *Dementia units in long-term care* (pp. 174–200). Baltimore: Johns Hopkins University Press.

Hiatt, L. G. (1991c). *Nursing home renovation.* Boston: Butterworth Heinman.

Hiatt, L. G. (1992). Restraint reduction with special emphasis on wandering behavior. *Topics in Geriatric Rehabilitation, 8*(2), 55–77.

Hiatt, L. G., Brandon, B., & Dunlap, R. (2001). 15 programming goals for successful dementia design. *Advances for Providers of Post-Acute Care, 4*(3), 44–50, 397–421.

Hoenig, H., Pieper, C., Zolkewitz, M., Schenkman, M., & Branch, L. G. (2002). Wheelchair users are not necessarily wheelchair bound. *Journal of American Geriatric Society, 50*(4), 771–772.

Hoglund, D., & Ledewitz, S. D. (1999). Designing to meet the needs of people with Alzheimer's disease. In B. Schwarz & R. Brent (Eds.), *Aging, autonomy, and architecture advances in assisted living* (pp. 229–261). Baltimore: Johns Hopkins.

Hope, T., Keene, J., Gedling, K., Fairburn, C. G., & Jacoby, R. (1998). Predictors of institutionalization for people with dementia living at home with a carer [*sic*]. *International Journal of Geriatric Psychiatry, 13*(10), 682–690.

Johnson, K. (1996). Exceptional staff. *Assisted Living Today, 3*(2), 5.

Kane, R. A., Caplan, A. L., Urv-Wong, E. K., Freeman, I. C., Aroskar, M. A., & Finch, M. (1997). Everyday matters in the lives of nursing home residents: Wish for and perception of choice and control. *Journal of the American Geriatrics Society, 45*(9), 1086–1093.

Kayser-Jones, J., & Schell, E. (1997). The effect of staffing on the quality of care at mealtime. *Nursing Outlook, 45,* 64–72.

Kayser-Jones, J., Schell, E., Lyons, W., Kris, A. E., Chan, J., & Beard, R. L. (2003). Factors that influence end-of-life care in nursing homes: The physical environment, inadequate staffing, and lack of supervision. *Gerontology, 43,* Special Issue 11, 76–84.

Kayser-Jones, J., Sobell, E. S., Porter, C., Barbaccia, J. C., & Shaw, H. (1998). Factors contributing to dehydration in nursing homes: Inadequate staffing and lack of professional supervision. *Journal of the American Geriatric Society, 7,* 1187–1194.

Kehoe, M. A., & Van Heesch, B. (in press). Culture change in long-term care: The Wellspring model. *Journal of Social Work in Long Term Care.*

Kendig, H. (2003). Directions in environmental gerontology: A multidisciplinary field. *Gerontologist, 43*(5), 611–614.

Kiely, D. K., Leveille, S. G., & Morris, J. N. (2002). Associating the onset of motor impairments with disability progression in nursing home residents. *American Journal of Physical Medicine and Rehabilitation, 81*(9), 696–704.

Kinkead, G. (2003, December 23). A room comes alive with color and sounds. *The New York Times,* p. F8.

Lawton, M. P., & Nahemow, L. (1973). Ecology and the aging process. In C. Eisdorfer and M. P. Lawton (Eds.), *The psychology of adult development and aging* (pp. 619–674). Washington, DC: American Psychological Association.

MacKenzie, S. (2003). Implementing the Eden Alternative in Australia. *Journal of Social Work in Long Term Care, 2*(1), 325–338.

Mahoney, D. F. (2003). Vigilance: Evolution and definition for caregivers of family members with Alzheimer's disease. *Journal of Gerontological Nursing, 29*(8), 24–30.

Marcus, C. C., & Barnes, M. (1999). *Healing gardens: Therapeutic benefits and design.* New York: John Wiley.

Marsden, J. P. (2001). A framework for understanding homelike character in the context of assisted living housing. *Journal of Housing for the Elderly, 15*(1/2), 79–96.

Mather, J. A., Nemecek, B. A., & Oliver, K. (1997). The effect of a walled garden on behavior of individuals with Alzheimer's. *American Journal of Alzheimer's Disease, 12*(6), 252–257.

Mikelson, P., & Johnson, J. (2003). Case study brief: The Lynblomstein Care Center, St. Paul, MN. *Journal of Social Work in Long Term Care, 2*(1), 301–306.

Mishima, M., Okawa, M. K., Hozami, S., & Hishikawa, Y. (2000). Supplementary administration of bright light and melatonin as potent treatment for disorganized circadian rest-activity and dysfunctional autonomic and neuroendocrine systems in institutionalized demented elderly persons. *Chronobiology International, 17*(3), 419–432.

Mollica, R. L. (1998). *State Assisted Living Policy, 1998. Executive summary.* Portland, ME: National Academy for State Health Policy. Available at http://nashp.org

Mollica, R. L., Wilson Brown, K., Ryther, B. S., & Lamarche, H. J. (1995). *Guide to assisted living and state policy.* Portland, ME: National Academy for State Health Policy.

Namazi, K. H., & Johnson, B. (2002). Pertinent autonomy for residents with dementias: Modification of the physical environment to enhance independence. *American Journal of Alzheimer's Care and Related Disorders and Research, 7*(1), 16–21.

Nolan, B. A. D., Mathews, R. M., & Harrison, M. (2001). Using external memory aids to increase room finding by older adults with dementia. *American Journal of Alzheimer's Disease and Other Dementias, 16*(4), 251–254.

Olsen, R., Hutchings, B. L., & Ehrenkrantz, E. (2000). "Media memory lane" interventions in an Alzheimer's day care center. *American Journal of Alzheimer's Care and Related Disorders & Research, 15*(3), 163–175.

Ouslander, J. G., Maloney, C., Grasela, T. H., Rogers, L., & Walawander, C. A. (2001). Implementation of a nursing home urinary incontinence management program with and without tolterodine. *Journal of the American Medical Directors Association, 2*(5), 207–214.

Pearson, A., Fitzgerald, M., & Nay, R. (2003). Mealtime in nursing homes: The role of nursing staff. *Journal of Gerontological Nursing, 29*(6), 41–44.

Perez, K., Proffitt, M. A., & Calkins, M. (2001). Minimizing disruptive behaviors. In *Creating successful dementia care settings, Vol 3.* Baltimore: Health Professionals Press.

Phillips, C. D., Sloane, P. D., Hawes, C. L., Koch, G., Hans, J. Spry, K., Duntemann, G., & Williams, R. I. (1997). Effects of residence in Alzheimer disease special care units on functional outcomes. *Journal of the American Medical Association, 278*(16), 1340–1344.

Pillemer, K. (1996). Eight myths about nursing assistant. *Contemporary Long Term Care, 19*(7), 44–46, 48, 52.

Reed, A. T., Lach, H. W., Smith, L., & Birge, S. J. (1990). Alzheimer's disease and the need for supervision. *American Journal of Alzheimer's Care and Related Disorders & Research, 14*, 29–34.

Remington, R. (2002). Calming music and hand massage with agitated elderly. *Nursing Research, 51*(5), 317–323.

Rosenfield, Z., & Wyatt, A. (1984). Urban nursing home rescued and renovated. *Hospitals, 58*(4), 109–110.

Sanford, J. A., & Megrew, M. B. (1995). An evaluation of grab bars to meet the needs of elderly people. *Assisted Technology, 7*(1), 36–47.

Schnelle, J. F., Cadogan, M. P., Grbic, D., Bates-Jensen, B. M., Osterweil, D., Yoshii, J., & Simmons, S. F. (2003). A standardized quality assessment system to evaluate incontinence care in the nursing home. *Journal of the American Geriatric Society, 51*(12), 1754–1761.

Schnelle, J. F., Cadogan, M. P., Yoshii, J., Al-Samarrai, N. R., Osterweil, D., Bates-Jensen, B. M., & Simmons, S. F. (2003). The minimum data set urinary incontinence quality indicators: Do they reflect differences in care processes related to incontinence? *Medical Care, 4,* 909–922.

Selvidge, M., Wylde, M., & Rummage, M. (1993). *Enabling products: A sourcebook.* Oxford, MS: Institute for Technology Development. Also available at 601-234-0158.

Sloane, P. (2001). *Bathing without battle.* New York: Springer.

Sloane, P. D., Linderman, D. A., Phillips, C., Morita, D. J., & Koch, G. (1995). Evaluating Alzheimer's special care units: Reviewing the evidence and identifying potential sources of study bias. *The Gerontologist, 35,* 103–111.

Society for the Advancement of Gerontological Environments (SAGE). (2003). SAGE brochure. 8055 Chardon Road, Kirtland, OH. Also available at www.SAGEFederation.com

Souder, E., & O'Sullivan, P. (2003). Disruptive behaviors of older adults in an institutional setting. *Journal of Gerontological Nursing, 29*(8), 31–36.

Stone, R. (2003). Selecting a model or choosing your own culture. *Journal of Social Work in Long Term Care, 2*(1), 411–422.

Thomas, W. H., & Johansson, C. (2003). Elderhood in Eden. *Topics in Geriatric Rehabilitation, 19*(4), 282–290.

Tofle, R. B., Schwarz, B., & Max-Royale, A. (2004). *Color in healthcare environments: A monograph reference guide.* Columbia, MO: Department of Environmental Design.

U.S. Centers for Medicare and Medicaid Services [CMS] (prepared by ABT Associates, Inc.) (2001). *Appropriateness of minimum nurse staffing ratios in nursing homes: Report to Congress: Phase II Final,* Vols. I–III. Baltimore: Author.

Valentine, N. M. (1998). Quality measures essential to the transformation of the Veterans Health Administration: Implications for nurses as co-creators of change. *Nurse Administration Quarterly, 22*(4), 76–87.

Vladeck, B. C. (1980). *Unloving care: The nursing home tragedy.* New York: Basic Books.

Voeks, S. K., Gallagher, C. M., Langer, E. H., & Drinka, P. J. (1990). Hearing loss in the nursing home. An institutional issue. *Journal of the American Geriatric Society, 38*(2), 141–145.

Wagner, J., & Creelman, D. (2004). A new image for long-term care. *Healthcare Finance Management, 58*(4), 70–74.

Wahl, H.-W., & Weisman, G. D. (2003). Environmental gerontology at the beginning of the new millennium: Reflections on its historical, empirical and theoretical development. *Gerontologist, 43,* Special Issue II, 616–627.

Walsh, B., Craik, K., & Price, R. H. (Eds.). (2000). *Person–environment psychology: New directions and perspectives.* Hillsdale, NJ: Erlbaum.

Werezak, L. J., & Morgan, D. G. (2003). Creating a therapeutic psychosocial environment in dementia care: A preliminary framework. *Journal of Gerontological Nursing, 29,* 12.

Whall, A. L., Black, M. E., Groh, C. J., Yankou, D. J., Kupferschmid, B. J., & Foster, N. J. (1997). The effect of natural environments upon agitation and aggression in late stage dementia patients. *American Journal of Alzheimer's Care and Related Disorders & Research, 12*(5), 216–217.

Wilkerson, D. L., & MacDonell, C. (2003). Quality oversight and culture change in long-term care. *Journal of Social Work in Long Term Care, 2*(1), 373–395.

Windley, P., & Scheidt, R. J. (1980). Person-environment dialects: Implications for competent functioning in old age. In L. W. Poon (Ed.), *Aging in the 1980s: Psychological issues.* Washington, DC: American Psychological Association.

Wylde, M. (1997, June). Traditional research doesn't account for all important features, expert says. *Housing The Elderly Report.*

Zimmerman, S., Gruber-Baldini, A. L., Sloane, P. D., Eckert, J. K., Hebel, J. R., Morgan, L. A., Stearns, S. C., Wildfire, J. W., Magaziner, J., Hyg, M. S., Chen, C., & Konrad, T. R. (2003). Assisted living and nursing homes: Apples and oranges? *Gerontologist, 43,* Special Issue II, 107–117.

# 5

# Home Health Care

## *Catherine DeLorey*

Home health care at the beginning of the twenty-first century is a microcosm of all that is both good and bad in our total health care system. It has highly dedicated and committed workers and organizations attempting to provide services in an imperfect system. Meanwhile, it is functioning in a morass of changing and cumbersome regulations within confusing reimbursement mechanisms.

Home care is a complex array of services ranging from assistance for activities of daily living to highly technical health care. Providers of these services range from informal, untrained family members to sophisticated, highly trained health care professionals. Perhaps the only underlying consistency is that these are health services offered outside an acute or long-term care facility.

Although many organizations, agencies, and health professionals are involved in providing home health care, it is essentially an issue of midlife and older women. The role of the untrained family member, most often a woman, in home health care is a major contribution to the services provided and, although difficult for the caregiver, provides a substantial financial savings in health care. More than 72% of informal caregivers are daughters or wives of home care patients, and women receive the bulk of long-term care services, including home health care (Health Resources and Services Administration, 2003b; Katz, Kabeto, & Langa, 2000; Levine, 1999).

This disparity not only impacts on women within the health care system, but has societal ramifications, as cited by Senator Hillary Rodham Clinton (Aging Subcommittee, 2002) in testimony before a joint senate committee:

1. Women outnumber men among the aging population. Thus women suffer disproportionately from our failure to develop a coherent long-

term care financing system, a problem exacerbated by the fact that older women are also twice as likely as men to live in a nursing home, and twice as likely to live in poverty.

2. An underlying reason our caregiving system is in disarray, and why these important functions are undervalued, underfinanced, and too often un-compensated in our society is because it was work that women performed in the homes. We too often take for granted the contribution that women made as caregivers. For too long, this work was "invisible," no one paid for it, and it didn't show up in the GDP.

3. Just because family caregiving is unpaid does not mean it is costless. The costs include not just time, and lost economic opportunities, but also personal strain and fatigue, and poor health. These costs should be recognized and this caregiver must be supported, through respite care and other services.

4. We are quickly realizing that our country is suffering not just from a budget deficit, but what has been called "a care deficit."

## MEDICARE'S ROLE IN HOME HEALTH CARE

Medicare was one of the most important entitlements of the Older Americans Act of 1966. However, in 1996 Medicare redefined home care to include only those selected functions and prescribed circum-stances that were reimbursable. It created a narrowly defined, frag-mented, and uncoordinated set of acute care services not well adapted to the chronically ill at home. Through Medicare, home health care was established as an alternative to institutional care. Therefore, service selection and delivery patterns were based on institutional patterns rather than as unique to the continuum of appropriate care for elders.

## THE HISTORY OF HOME HEALTH CARE

To begin to understand the complexities of home health care today, we must first visit its interesting and varied history. We will see that home health care did not grow out of perceived need and then plan to meet that need. Instead, it developed out of an array of motivations, from the benevolent wealthy women of the nineteenth century, to health departments, voluntary agencies, and insurance companies with their own incentives. This led to a great deal of overlap in services and a strange amalgam of means to finance these services. Throughout this history, the goals and functions of home health care have changed as those who managed and paid for it determined what it is (Rosen, 1993). We have yet to overcome this legacy.

We will focus on how home health care has been provided to all persons, not just to older persons, because the history of home health care is rich, complex, and reflective of the social history of each era surrounding it, not just to the elderly. Knowing this history helps us to understand the roads home health care has traveled, and gives us insight into where it may be going. Putting elders into the picture expands the complexity and highlights the ambivalence of what home health care is, or should be.

Home health care has existed for millennia but its contemporary path parallels that of increased urbanization and the development of the profession of nursing. At the beginning of the nineteenth century, home health care was a part of familial life. The person with medical needs was cared for by family, servants, or neighbors. However, for those without such resources, there were few options.

It is from an observation of this condition that one of the first formal home care providers, the Ladies Benevolent Society of Charleston, South Carolina, focused on caring for the sick at home. At mid-century, both in the north and south of the Untied States, upper-class, affluent women, also known as "Lady Bountifuls," worked together to address the social needs of their communities. This naturally led them to the dilemma of caring for the homebound sick who hired other women to provide services. Yet even then, need was always greater than available resources.

From the beginning there were questions concerning who should be the recipients of care. This reflects the conundrum in all of social welfare services at that the time—who were the "worthy poor." The Ladies Benevolent Society continued until the end of the century, constantly dealing with how to pay for services, what services to offer, and to whom.

As immigration to the United States increased and cities enlarged, affluent women in the north also took up the challenge of providing care for the poor sick in the cities. By this time they were impressed with the British model of providing trained nurses to visit in the homes to give care. Thus began the Visiting Nurse Associations (VNA).

Through the end of the nineteenth century and the beginning of the twentieth, VNAs developed as voluntary, women-dominated organizations. Yet as these organizations and their scope grew, they needed more professional management. The women leaders of the VNAs complemented their managerial skills and supplemented their own financial contributions through fundraising activities and solicitations among their peers. This growth and development of the voluntary VNAs became the initial expression of formal home health care in the United States.

Trained nurses in the home focused on providing direct care, including dealing with contagious illnesses. Because most of this care was to the evolving and revolving poor, immigrant communities, the role of the trained nurse grew into that of health educator and caregiver. The trained nurses were for the poor and dealt primarily with the dangerously ill, that is, persons with communicable diseases. These people attracted the attention of benefactors and caregiving organizations. The "uninteresting sick" were those persons with chronic diseases, who at that time were seen only as passive individuals needing nothing more than custodial care. Lillian Wald, a graduate nurse from an affluent New York family, was the first to coin the phrase "public health nurse," after visiting some neighborhoods on the lower east side of New York City. She saw the squalor and illnesses there as a breakdown of society's infrastructure, not just the impact of contaminants or bacteria.

Although the voluntary agencies were effective, advances in technology in the mid-1900s gradually made care in an institutional setting more economical, and home care became less popular. It continued to diminish with the boom of employer-paid health benefits during World War II.

As home care organizations developed, other players entered the arena. In addition to the voluntary organizations, private groups and health departments sprang up. This was not necessarily a positive development as home health care evolved to be responsive to social changes rather than becoming a leader in determining how to meet health needs outside of institutions. This unbridled growth became so uncoordinated that by 1909, in New York City, there were 58 organizations that sent out 372 nurses (Buhler-Wilkerson, 2001).

Health departments, by statute, are responsible for the general health of the community and concerned with prevention of disease and health promotion. Because there were no societal regulations or formal planning for development of the home health care industry, the unchecked growth of agencies led to an overlap of responsibilities among voluntary, private, and public organizations.

Because of the formal role of health departments, one of the unintended consequences of the increased use of nurses by health departments was that publicly supported nurses were seen to be for prevention, and home care of the sick was left to the voluntary agencies, or VNAs. This dichotomy is still prevalent.

By 1911 a new era was evolving in home care. The Metropolitan Life Insurance Company was convinced that providing for nurses to visit in the home would be cost saving for the company. The rationale was that it would save the insurance company revenues by keeping people healthier through the intervention of public health nurses. This was a forward thinking and dynamic program. But as hospital growth increased and it seemed that home visits were not financially profitable, Metropolitan Life Insurance slowly exited its home care services.

Although home care generally decreased during the 1940s, it was at this time that Montefiore Medical Center in the Bronx, New York, began its "hospital without walls" program. Physicians, nurses, and other clinical professionals successfully administered care to community residents in their homes, and the program ultimately served as a model for modern home health agencies.

The uncharted growth of health care agencies continued, so that by the 1950s there was a patchwork of funding mechanisms, including:

1.  Community Chests (United Way), providing 44% of home health care costs
2.  Private patient fees, providing 16% of home health care costs
3.  Municipal funds, providing 15% of home health care costs
4.  Private contributions, providing 10% of home health care costs
5.  Public welfare, including Veterans Administration, providing 15% of home health care costs

As with all aspects of health care, home health care has influenced and been influenced by larger societal trends and social history. Its roles and functions have evolved through the constant pull of economic and social trends.

These trends have included the ambivalence in United States culture between individual and community responsibility. This was a conflict at the time of the Ladies Benevolent Society and it continues today. Who are the worthy sick and who is not deserving of society's beneficence? How do we decide what to pay for, how much to pay, and what we will ask the individual to pay?

With the advent of Medicare in 1966, home care began to gain momentum. By the end of the 1980s, the number of Medicare-certified home care agencies had tripled (Gundersen, 1999). Home health care has gone in and out of favor, but in all its iterations it has never really been defined and lacks a distinct identity that describes it in more than the obverse of other types of health care.

## HOME HEALTH CARE DEFINED

In its simplest definition, home health care is health care offered in the home. But there the simplicity stops. It is actually more than health care—it is a full range of services, intended to keep the individual as healthy as possible in the non-institutional setting.

Because we are focusing on the older population, we will only address home health care as it relates to older persons, but we cannot lose sight of the fact that it is offered to individuals of all ages, from the infant sent home with a major congenital anomaly who needs habilitation, to the young person who has a bullet lodged in the spine, to the person with a chronic condition needing ongoing care, from persons who are post-operative, to persons receiving rehabilitative care, to persons receiving maintenance care for chronic disease conditions, and to persons receiving end-of-life care through home hospice, which will be discussed in chapter 11.

The wide range of services can include personal care like bathing, toileting, and dressing. It can include highly skilled care with complex medical procedures, similar to those received at acute care facilities, such as kidney dialysis (Calkins, Boult, Wagner, & Pacala, 1999; Campion, 1995). These services are delivered at home to recovering, disabled, and chronically or terminally ill persons in need of medical, nursing, social, or therapeutic treatment, and/or assistance with the essential activities of daily living. One could even consider care offered in an assisted living facility as home health care because it is care given in the resident's home, not offered by the institution.

Aging brings many changes for our parents and grandparents. Most important among these changes is the fight for independence as they may lose the ability to drive, enjoy hobbies, see, hear, or simply complete daily activities of living. However, in planning for retirement, older people tend to focus their efforts on financial, legal, and estate issues. What are often mistakenly overlooked are the issues of housing and care. These needs are often left until a medical trauma occurs and, as a result, we are forced to make uninformed care decisions with considerable pressure and speed. These decisions can seriously impact a caregiver's life. A national survey conducted by the National Alliance for Caregiving/AARP (American Association of Retired Persons, 2002) provides some insight into how family caregivers lives are influenced by these responsibilities. These influences included:

- Two in 10 working caregivers turned down chances to work on special projects; almost as many avoided work-related travel
- Forty percent of the survey respondents said that caregiving affected their ability to advance in their jobs
- Twenty-nine percent passed up a job promotion, training, or assignment

- Twenty-five percent passed up an opportunity for a job transfer or relocation
- Twenty-two percent were not able to acquire new job skills.

These decisions may seriously impact a caregiver's life.

Generally, home care is appropriate for a person who needs ongoing care that cannot easily or effectively be provided solely by family and friends, but does not need to be in a hospital or other facility. More and more older people, electing to live independent, non-institutionalized lives, are receiving home care services as their physical capabilities diminish. (Fried, van Doorn, O'Leary, Tinetti, & Drickamer, 2000; Gundersen, 1999; Naylor, Brooten, Jones, Lavizzo-Mourey, Mezey, & Pauly, 1994; O'Leary, Tinetti, & Drickamer, 1999). As hospital stays decrease, increasing numbers of patients need highly skilled services when they return home. Other patients are able to stay at home to begin with, receiving safe and effective care.

Although Medicare changed the definition of home health care to an alternative to institutional care, rather than a service in its own right, providers of home care have continued to abide by the principles of public health prevention while providing their services in an ever changing health care environment (Welch, Wennberg, & Welch, 1996). Older persons with health conditions serious enough to warrant home health care do not just receive custodial, unplanned care.

## HEALTH PROMOTION: PRIMARY, SECONDARY, AND TERTIARY PREVENTION

In addition to acute health services, care is provided that includes the three levels of prevention basic to any public health practice. Primary, secondary, and tertiary prevention are as relevant to care for older persons with chronic conditions as in any other health care domain. Health promotion and disease prevention improve the health status of older persons without increasing the costs in the long run (Lubitz, Liming, Kramarow, & Lentzner, 2003).

Primary prevention is intervention or care provided to individuals to prevent the onset of a condition (U.S. Preventive Services Task Force, 2002). This can include health education, health communication, social marketing to prevent or stop smoking, and interventions such as immunizations. In home care for elders these activities could consist of the provider recommending flu or pneumonia immunizations, education to the client and family on appropriate nutrition, or safety factors in the home.

Secondary prevention measures are those that identify and treat persons who have developed risk factors or preclinical disease but in whom the condition may not be clinically apparent. These activities focus on early case findings to avoid further complications. Screening tests are examples of secondary prevention activities. With early case finding, the natural history of disease, or how the course of an illness unfolds, can often be altered to maximize well-being and minimize suffering. In the arena of elder home care, examples of these interventions are screening for anemia, diabetes, or hypercholesteremia and providing appropriate counsel. A very important role of the nurse giving care in the home is anticipatory guidance. Because nurses are really caring for the whole family unit, not just the elder client, they can anticipate issues that might arise and help the family and client prepare for them. Palliative care and issues of death and dying are significant tasks to help families prepare in a manner appropriate for all.

Tertiary prevention activities involve the care of established disease, with attempts made to restore the client to highest possible function, minimize the negative effects of disease, and prevent disease-related complications. The aim of tertiary prevention in older people is to identify and alleviate established disease at an early stage in order to improve or maintain functional status. The rationale depends on the ability to prevent disability and handicap, but not necessarily the impairment itself, which may not be amenable to a specific treatment. Unreported need plus multiple pathology and morbidity have a cumulative effect, so where one problem might be relatively minor, the cumulative effect of several problems may result in loss of function (e.g., poor mobility) and reduction in quality of life.

## THE DEMOGRAPHICS OF HOME HEALTH CARE

Chapter 1 of this book introduced the reader to the demographics of aging: persons 65 years and older now account for 35 million of the population; by 2030, the older population will number over 70 million (Tepper, this volume). The over-65 population is steadily growing, and it will continue its upward pattern in the coming years. Medical advances, preventive care, and a greater understanding of the benefits of a healthy lifestyle have contributed to an increase in the average life expectancy. Upon reaching the age of 65, males may expect to live an additional

16.3 years, and women, 19.2 years (Administration on Aging 2002). This increased longevity has major implications for families and society.

As people age, chances increase that they will develop a chronic condition or a physical or cognitive disability for which they will require assistance. For example, 47% of individuals 50–64 years of age have some type of chronic condition but no disability, whereas 83% of individuals 85 years of age and older live simultaneously with chronic conditions, disability, and accompanying functional limitations.

## WHO ARE RECIPIENTS OF CARE?

The aging baby boomer generation will soon be more than a prediction, and family members, who often provide at least a portion of care to their aging relatives, may often be unprepared to deal with the many issues facing both them and the senior. From planning a change of residence to communicating effectively, there are many simple, yet often overlooked ways to ease caregiving for the elderly and their family members when home care is needed.

Deciding what services are needed and how they will be provided is a complex question, depending where the person sits on the continuum of need, as well as what social supports and family resources are available (Lieberman, 2000). A person living alone without social or family support will need intervention more than the person with strong supports. This is one reason that women require more health care supports as they age; they have often taken care of a spouse who may have died, or the spouse may not be able to take on the required responsibilities.

An increasing number of individuals are receiving health care at home or in community-based settings rather than in institutions. In 2000, 1,355,300 Americans received home health care services. Of these, females comprised 877,900 (64.8%) of recipients. The majority of women receiving home health care were aged 65 years or older (76.1%). Women aged 85 and older received 25.6% of home health care, followed by women between the ages of 75 and 79 (18.4%) (HRSA, 2003a).

In 2000, 73.2% of female and 78.3% of male home health care patients received skilled nursing services. Additional services commonly provided to home health patients include personal care, physical therapy, and homemaker household services (HRSA, 2003b).

Increasing numbers of women and men are turning to hospice care to meet their end-of-life needs. Between 1992 and 2000, the number of hospice care patients increased from 52,000 to 105,500. Women narrowly outnumbered men in the number of hospice care patients, comprising 53.5% of patients in 1992 and 57.4% of patients in 2000 (HRSA, 2003a).

## SERVICE PROVIDERS IN HOME HEALTH CARE

Home health care agencies provide much of the care to older people in the community. Some are private, profit-making organizations, and some are non-profit. They provide services such as meals, nursing care (RNs, LPNs, CNAs, and home health aides), occupational therapy, and physical therapy. Community health nurses provide a majority of care. This type of care requires a specialized health care professional.

One of the major characterizations for health professionals doing home health care is that they are not in a clinical setting where they are surrounded by a system of professional and mechanical resources. The home health care worker is a guest in the patient's home. Home is the patient's domain, not the health worker's.

Home health care is available through hospitals, agencies, and public health departments. It encompasses services provided by nurses, therapists, and aides, including:

1. Health care such as nursing, social work, physical and rehabilitative therapy, medication monitoring, and medical equipment
2. Personal care such as assistance with hygiene, dressing, bathing, and exercise
3. Nutrition, including meal planning, cooking, and meal delivery
4. Homemaking, including housekeeping, shopping, and household paperwork
5. Social and safety needs such as transportation services, companions, and a daily telephone check

In 1997, at least 52 million people in the United States provided informal or unpaid care for family members or friends (National Alliance for Caregiving 1997). Estimates put the value of unpaid care annually at $196 billion (Arno, Levine, & Memmott, 1999; Emanuel, Fairclough, Slutsman, & Emanuel, 2000). As important and rewarding as caring for family or friends might be, paid home care services may also be required to supplement informal care because of the caregiver's work responsibilities, geographic distance, or the caregiver's own limitations. In 1998, formal, or paid, home care services were used by 28% of individuals aged 50–64 years who required help with activities of daily living. Only nine percent of the same age group used unpaid home care services. In the same year, the greatest increase in use of paid home care occurred in the 75–84-year-old age bracket. Forty eight percent of this older age group used paid home care and 26% used unpaid care (Gibson, 2003).

## PROGRAM OF ALL INCLUSIVE CARE
## FOR THE ELDERLY (PACE)

The PACE programs grew out of the On Lok model of providing health care to frail elders, created in San Francisco in 1971. On Lok means "peaceful, happy abode" in Cantonese (Bodenheimer, 1999). PACE is unique. It is an optional benefit under both Medicare and Medicaid that focuses entirely on older people who are frail enough to meet their state's standards for nursing home care (Centers for Medicare & Medicaid Services, 2003a) and features comprehensive medical and social services. PACE permits most patients to continue living at home while receiving services rather than being institutionalized. A team of doctors, nurses, and other health professionals assess participant needs, develop care plans, and deliver all services, which are integrated into a complete health care plan. Because PACE clients must meet the requirements for nursing home care, many states support its services under their Medicaid programs. Eligible individuals who wish to participate must voluntarily enroll. To be eligible, a person must be at least 55 years of age; live in the PACE service area; be screened by a team of doctors, nurses, and other health professionals; and sign and consent to the terms of the enrollment agreements.

PACE offers and manages all of the medical, social, and rehabilitative services enrollees need to preserve or restore their independence, to remain in their homes and communities, and to maintain their quality of life. The PACE service package must include all Medicare and Medicaid services provided by the state. In addition, there are an additional 16 home or long term care facility services that a PACE organization must provide, including social work, medication, and nursing facility care. Minimum services that must be provided in the PACE center include primary care services, social services, restorative therapies, personal care and supportive services, nutritional counseling, recreational therapy, meals, and transportation. Services are available 24 hours a day, 7 days a week, and 365 days a year. Generally, these services are provided in an adult day health center setting, but may also include in-home and other referral services that enrollees may need. This includes medical specialists, laboratory and other diagnostic services, and hospital and nursing home care.

An enrollee's need is determined by PACE's medical team of care providers. PACE teams include primary care physicians and nurses; physical, occupational, and recreational therapists; social workers; personal care attendants; dietitians; and drivers. Generally, the PACE team has daily contact with enrollees. This helps them detect subtle changes in enrollees' conditions and enables them to react quickly to changing medical, functional, and psychosocial needs.

## HOSPICE AND HOME HEALTH CARE

A hospice is a facility that provides inpatient, outpatient, or home care for the terminally ill person. This care is palliative, not focused on attempting to cure a condition but intended to provide a positive end-of-life experience for the client and family by alleviating pain, dealing with symptoms, and making the person as comfortable as possible (Pearson & Stubbs, 1999; Schultz et al., 2003).

When Congress passed TEFRA (the Tax Equity and Fiscal Responsibility Act) in 1982, it created a Medicare hospice benefit (PL 97-248). Hospice services may be provided to terminally ill Medicare beneficiaries with a life expectancy of six months or less, if the disease runs its normal course.

Effective with the enactment of the Balanced Budget Act of 1997 (PL 105-33) (Social Security Online, 2003), the Medicare hospice benefit was divided into the following periods: (1) an initial 90-day period, (2) a subsequent 90-day period, and (3) an unlimited number of subsequent 60-day benefit periods as long as the patient continues to meet program eligibility requirements. The beneficiary must be recertified as terminally ill at the beginning of each benefit period. The following covered hospice services are provided as necessary to give palliative treatment for conditions related to the terminal illness:

- nursing care
- services of a medical social worker
- physician care
- counseling (including dietary, pastoral, and other)
- home care aide and homemaker
- short-term inpatient care (including both respite care and inpatient care for pain control and acute and chronic system management)

- medical appliances and supplies (including drugs and biologicals)
- physical and occupational therapies
- speech and language pathology services
- bereavement service for the family up to 13 months following the patient's death

Medicare hospice participation has grown at a dramatic rate, largely as a result of a 1989 Congressional mandate (PL 101-239) that increased rates by 20%. From 1984 to January 2002, the total number of hospices participating in Medicare rose from 31 to 2,265—more than a 73-fold increase. Of these hospices, 1,003 are freestanding, 690 are home health agency-based, 552 are hospital-based, and 20 are skilled nursing facility-based (National Association for Homecare and Hospice, 2002).

## HOME HEALTH CARE AGENCY CERTIFICATION

For an agency to receive Medicare reimbursement it must be certified by the Centers for Medicaid and Medicare Services (CMS) (Health Care Financing Administration, 1998). The Outcome and Assessment Information Set (OASIS), the primary method used by Medicare to certify home health agencies, is a group of data elements that represent core items of a comprehensive assessment for an adult home care patient. In addition, it forms the basis for measuring patient outcomes for purposes of outcome-based quality improvement (OBQI).

The OASIS is a key component of Medicare's partnership with the home care industry to foster and monitor improved home health care outcomes and is proposed to be an integral part of the revised Conditions of Participation for Medicare-certified home health agencies (HHA).

Most data items in the OASIS were derived in the context of a CMS-funded national research program to develop a system of outcome measures for home health care. Overall, the OASIS items are useful for outcome monitoring, clinical assessment, care planning, and other internal agency-level applications (CMS, 2003b).

## PAYING FOR HOME HEALTH CARE

The crazy quilt of reimbursement mechanisms and regulations in home health care reflects what occurs in the larger health care system, but in reality are magnified. As we saw in the discussion of the origins of home health care, it has been responsive to community needs rather than proactive. This results in a service that is constantly changing to meet external forces, rather than the needs of the constituency it serves.

The complexities of deciding how we will pay for home care is a dilemma of economic, professional, and social value issues. We need to answer questions that reflect these values:

1.  When does a person need professional, formal home health care?
2.  When does the individual no longer need home health care?
3.  What can our expectations of improvement be?
4.  How are we going to pay for this service and who should pay for it?
5.  Is this appropriate, realistic, and cost-effective for both the client and society?

## MECHANISMS FOR PAYMENT

Although Medicare is the major player in the reimbursement game for persons over 65 years of age, there are other options for payment of home health care services. These include private payers, Medigap insurance, both private and public, and payment through long-term care insurance.

### Private Pay

Although not used exclusively (except by those with adequate financial resources), with the various mechanisms of co-payments, deductibles, and co-insurance most older persons make a substantial contribution of their own finances to their health care and home care. Insurance experts estimate that about one-third of all long-term care services are paid for by individuals out of their own savings or investments. The funds may come from pension plans, employee stock ownership plans, single premium annuities, the cash value of life insurance, or savings (MetLife, 2003).

### Long-Term Care Insurance

This is private insurance designed to help pay for nursing home or home health care expenses. It is available to individuals and may be available under a group policy. The insured pays a premium to an insurer in return for protection against the high costs of long-term care (Mature Market Institute, 2003; McCullough & Wilson, 1995).

Home health care services typically covered by long-term care insurance include nursing care, therapy, personal care, and homemaking. Generally, home health care agencies and providers must be state licensed or certified. Most policies contain a waiting period during which no benefits are paid. After the person has satisfied the waiting period, the policy pays up to a maximum dollar amount for each day of approved care. A policy may not cover all expenses.

Many policies now offer an inflation adjustment feature that increases the per-day benefit to cover higher costs. Premiums for long-term care insurance can vary widely, depending upon age and the level of benefits. The older a person is when first buying a long-term care policy, the higher the premiums probably will be because the probability of needing long-term care increases with age.

**Medicare**

There are strict eligibility roles for home health benefits (Medicare Rights Center, 2003). Medicare pays if care is provided by a Medicare-certified home agency and the person requires skilled nursing care, physical therapy, or speech therapy. A physician must regularly review the care plan and verify that the patient is homebound (Palmer, 2003).

People who qualify for home care reimbursement, which means that they require intermittent, highly skilled technical care, can have access to physical therapy, occupational therapy, speech therapy, medical social services, home health aides, and durable medical equipment such as hospital beds and oxygen.

Hospice benefits are in their own category, with services limited to 210 days, as a requirement for hospice services is that the patient will live no longer than six months. Medicare hospice payment covers all the services for general home care in addition to a contribution of 5% or $5.00 toward each prescription.

The major gaps in Medicare's long-term coverage are:

- No coverage for custodial care, either at home or in a nursing home
- No coverage in a nursing home without prior hospitalization
- No coverage for nursing home care after 100 days
- Coverage only in a Medicare-approved facility

With the enactment of the Balanced Budget Act of 1997, Congress approved the most far-reaching reforms in the 34-year history of Medicare—some 300 provisions that added even more complexity to the program. In the process, Congress greatly expanded the responsibilities of the HCFA and the Medicare Payment Advisory Commission, which it created to monitor the administration of the program. The reforms were intended to expand the choices among private health plans that beneficiaries may select by creating the new "Medicare+Choice" program and to strengthen Medicare's finances by including policies further constraining payments to providers in the traditional fee-for-service program and in managed-care plans (Iglehart, 1999).

To constrain Medicare home health spending growth, the Balanced Budget Act (BBA) of 1997 replaced Medicare's cost-based, per-visit payment method with a prospective payment system (PPS) by fiscal year 2000. Until PPS could be implemented, BBA imposed spending controls under an interim payment system.

For three years beginning October 1, 1997, the interim payment system incorporated tighter per-visit cost limits than had previously been in place and subjected each home health agency to an annual Medicare revenue cap, which was the product of an agency-specific, per-beneficiary amount and the number of beneficiaries that the home health agency served (General Accounting Office, 2002).

## Medicare Supplement Insurance

Often called Medigap, this is private insurance that supplements Medicare benefits and may cover co-payments and deductibles for medical and hospital expenses. Medigap policies generally do not provide coverage for long-term care. The Medicare benefit package is inadequate because it leaves beneficiaries liable for nearly half the cost of their acute care. In addition to deductibles, beneficiaries must pay 20 percent of their physicians' fees; there is no annual cap on the amount. Because of these high out-of-pocket expenses, 85 percent of beneficiaries have supplemental insurance (Moon, 2001).

## Medicaid

A joint federal/state program, Medicaid pays for health care for people with limited income and assets. It is often used as medi-gap insurance for those who cannot afford private insurance. To receive Medicaid, individuals must meet federal poverty guidelines for income and assets and may have to "spend down" or use up most of their assets. Some assets, such as a home, may not be counted when determining Medicaid eligibility.

## Medicare Managed Care

Instead of purchasing a Medigap policy, some people enroll in a Medicare HMO to supplement their Medicare benefits. Such plans may provide more preventive services and charge lower co-payments. However, one is generally restricted to participating providers (physicians, hospitals, nursing homes, etc.). Short-term nursing home care covered by Medicare and Medicare HMO is usually available only in participating facilities.

## PACE

PACE is the unique program that provides home care to frail elders and receives a fixed monthly payment per enrollee from Medicare and Medicaid. The amounts are the same during the contract year, regardless of the services an enrollee may need. Persons enrolled in PACE also may have to pay a monthly premium, depending on their eligibility for Medicare and Medicaid.

## CONCLUSION

This discussion has presented many of the complexities and frustrations of home health care, from its myriad reimbursement mechanisms to its plethora of service regulations. In a perfect world we would have services and payment designed to meet the health needs of older persons wherever they are on the health care continuum. Until that time, health providers and agencies will work within an imperfect system to provide the best care possible. Home health care reflects values of the larger society—how it thinks health care should be provided, who should receive health care, and how it values its elder population.

As a result of escalating aging populations, the spread of communicable disease, threats of bio-terrorism and war, and access to basic resources, care around the world is shifting from management of acute illness to chronic illness. Management of long-term chronic conditions requires coordinated community-based planning and strategies. Home care, hospice, and palliative care are best equipped to meet these changing needs. They will evolve to be the core of health care and social services in the coming decades.

## REFERENCES

Administration on Aging. (2002). *A profile of older Americans: 2002.* Available at http://www.aoa.dhhs.gov/prof/Statistics/statistics.asp

Aging Subcommittee. (2002). *Women and aging: Bearing the burden of long term care.* Available at http://aging.senate.gov/events/hr76hc.htm

American Association of Retired Persons (AARP). (2002). *Family caregiving and long term care.* Available at: http://research.aarp.org/il/fs91_ltc.html#pdf

Arno, P. S., Levine, C., & Memmott, M. M. (1999). The economic value of informal caregiving. *Health Affairs, 18*(2), 182–188.

Bodenheimer, T. (1999). Long term care for frail elderly people: The On Lok model. *New England Journal of Medicine, 341*(17), 1324–1328.

Buhler-Wilkerson, K. (2001). *No place like home: A history of nursing and home care in the United States.* Baltimore: Johns Hopkins University Press.

Calkins, E., Boult, C., Wagner, E. H., & Pacala, J. T. (1999). *New ways to care for older people: Building systems based on evidence.* New York: Springer.

Campion, E. W. (1995). New hope for home care? (Editorial). *New England Journal of Medicine, 333*(18), 1213–1214.

Centers for Medicare & Medicaid Services (CMS). (2003a). *Program of all inclusive care for the elderly (PACE).* Available at http://www.medicare.gov/Nursing/Alternatives/Pace.asp

Centers for Medicaid and Medicare Services (CMS). (2003b). *OASIS overview.* Available at http://www.cms.gov/oasis/hhoview.asp

Emanuel, E. J., Fairclough, D. L., Slutsman, J., & Emanuel, L. L. (2000). Understanding economic and other burdens of terminal illness: The experience of patients and their caregivers. *Annals of Internal Medicine, 132*(6), 451–459.

Fried, T. R., van Doorn, C., O'Leary, J. R., Tinetti, M. E., & Drickamer, A. (2000). Older persons' preference for home vs hospital care in the treatment of acute illness. *Archives of Internal Medicine, 160,* 1501–1506.

General Accounting Office (GAO). (2002). *Report to congressional committees—Medicare home health care—payments to home health agencies are considerably higher than costs.* Washington, DC: Author.

Gibson, M. J. (2003). *A report to the nation on independent living and disability.* Washington, DC: American Association of Retired Persons.

Gundersen, L. (1999). There's no place like home: The home health care alternative. *Annals of Internal Medicine, 131*(8), 639–640.

Health Care Financing Administration (HRSA). (1998). *Medicare memo: HCPCS requirements.* Milwaukee, WI: United Government Services, LLC.

Health Resources and Services Administration (HRSA), Maternal and child health. (2003a). *Home Health and Hospice Care.* Available at http://www.hsrnet.com/pubs/whusa03/pages/page_74.htm

Health Resources and Services Administration (HRSA). (2003b). *Women's health USA 2003.* Available at http://www.hsrnet.com/pubs/whusa03/pages/page_03.htm

Iglehart, J. K. (1999). The American health care system: Medicare. *New England Journal of Medicine, 340*(4), 327–332.

Katz, S. J., Kabeto, M., & Langa, K. M. (2000). Gender disparities in the receipt of home care for elderly people with disability in the United States. *Journal of the American Medical Association, 284,* 3022–3027.

Levine, C. (1999). The loneliness of the long-term caregiver. *New England Journal of Medicine, 340*(20), 1587–1590.

Lieberman, T. (2000). *Complete guide to health services for seniors.* New York: Three Rivers.

Lubitz, J., Liming, D., Kramarow, E., & Lentzner, H. (2003). Health, life expectancy, and health care spending among the elderly. *New England Journal of Medicine, 349*(11), 1048–1055.

Mature Market Institute. (2003). *The Metlife market survey of nursing home and home health care costs.* Westport, CT: MetLife Mature Market Institute.

McCullough, L. B., & Wilson, N. L. (Eds.). (1995). *Long term care decisions: Ethical and conceptual dimensions.* Baltimore: Johns Hopkins University Press.

Medicare Rights Center. (2003). *To obtain the Medicare home health benefit.* Available at http://www.medicarerights.org/maincontentobtaininghomecare.html

MetLife Mature Market Institute. (2003). *Long term care—Who pays for long term care?* Available at http://www.metlife.com/Applications/Corporate/WPS/CDA/PageGenerator/0,1674,P1863,00.html

Moon, M. (2001). Medicare. *New England Journal of Medicine, 344*(12), 928–931.

National Alliance for Caregiving. (1997). *Family caregiving in the U.S.: Findings from a national survey.* Washington DC: Author.

Naylor, M., Brooten, D., Jones, R., Lavizzo-Mourey, R., Mezey, M., & Pauly, M. (1994). Comprehensive discharge planning for the hospitalized elderly: A randomized clinical trial. *Annals of Internal Medicine, 120*(12), 999–1006.

National Association for Homecare and Hospice. (2002). *2002 hospice statistics.* Available at http://www.nahc.org/consumer/hpstats

O'Leary, J. R., Tinetti, M. E., & Drickamer, M. A. (1999). Older persons' preferences for site of terminal care. *Annals of Internal Medicine, 131*(2), 109–112.

Palmer, E. (2003). The Tower of Babel: A physician's guide to home care terminology. *The Journal of Home Care Medicine, 10*(1), 10.

Pearson, C., & Stubbs, M. L. (1999). *Parting company: Understanding the loss of a loved one—the caregiver's journey.* Seattle: Seal.

Rosen, G. (1993). *A history of public health.* Baltimore: Johns Hopkins University Press.

Schultz, R., Mendelsohn, A. B., Haley, W. E., Mahoney, D., Allen, R. S., Zhang, S., Thompson, L., & Belle, S. H. (2003). End-of-life care and the effects of bereavement on family caregivers of persons with dementia. *New England Journal of Medicine, 349*(20), 1936–1942.

Social Security Online. (2003). *Balanced Budget Act of 1997—P.L. 105-33,* Approved August 5, 1997 (111 Stat. 329). Available at http://www.ssa.gov/OP_Home/comp2/F105-033.html

U.S. Preventive Services Task Force. (2002). *Guide to clinical preventive services: Report of the U.S. Preventive Services Task Force* (3rd ed.). Alexandria, VA: International Medical Publishers.

Welch, H. G., Wennberg, D. E., & Welch, W. P. (1996). The use of Medicare home health care services. *New England Journal of Medicine, 335*(5), 324–329.

Wenger, N. S., Solomon, D. H., Roth, C. P., MacLean, C. H., Saliba, D., Kamberg,
    C. J., Rubenstein, L. Z., Young, R. T., Sloss, E. M., Louie, R., Adams, J., Chang,
    J. T., Venus, P. J. Schnelle, J. F., & Shekelle, P. G. (2003). The quality of medical
    care provided to vulnerable community-dwelling older patients. *Annals of Internal
    Medicine, 139*(9), 740–747.

# Part II

Health and Wellness
in Later Life

# 6

# Medical Care of the Elderly

## Richard H. Rubin

G eriatric medicine encompasses those areas relevant to the health care of the elderly, including diagnosis, treatment, and prevention. In addition to referring to a specific (and ever-expanding) body of knowledge, geriatric medicine features an approach to the patient that differs in several notable respects from the approach to younger adults.

Although practitioners of various types have provided health care to society's elders since the dawn of medicine, geriatric medicine per se is actually a rather new specialty. Training programs (termed fellowships) in geriatric medicine have been in existence since the 1970s. In 1988, two leading oversight organizations in medical education, the American Board of Internal Medicine and the American Board of Family Practice, agreed to jointly sponsor an examination that would provide certification to those clinicians who had attained a high level of expertise in the diagnosis and management of medical problems in the elderly. In the United States, health care for older persons is currently delivered by a mix of clinicians, primarily family medicine physicians and internists (those who specialize in the care of adults). In addition, a variety of other clinicians, including physician-assistants and nurse-practitioners, also provide care to many elders nationwide.

Chapter 1 in this text has underscored a number of demographic facts and projections crucial to geriatricians (physicians who specialize in the care of the elderly). Especially noteworthy is the increasing percentage of the U.S. population 65 years of age and older. In 1950, for example, 8.2% of the U.S. population was 65 or older. By the year 2000, that percentage had grown to 12.6%. Furthermore, it is estimated that by the year 2050 that figure will increase to 20.3% (Fowles & Greenberg, 2001). Because the elderly utilize health care services at a greater rate than younger persons, this demographic shift will likely have a major effect on health care financing and delivery in the United States (Spillman & Lubitz, 2000).

Given the breadth of geriatric medicine, this chapter will focus on several key issues:

- Normal aging versus pathology
- Common medical problems in the elderly
- Diagnostic challenges in the elderly (including atypical presentation of disease)
- Approach to the elderly patient

## NORMAL AGING VERSUS PATHOLOGY

### Case 1

*Ms. Adams is a 74-year-old retired kindergarten teacher in good general health who slipped on a patch of ice while walking her dog, landing squarely on her lower back. Because of persistent pain unrelieved by over-the-counter medication, she sees her physician, Dr. Baker, the following afternoon. Dr. Baker, concerned that the fall may have caused a vertebral (spine) fracture, recommends lumbosacral (low back) x-rays for Ms. Adams. The x-rays show no fracture but do show evidence of osteoarthritis (that is, "wear-and-tear" arthritic changes) as well as osteopenia (decreased bone density). Ms. Adams asks Dr. Baker if these x-ray findings are normal or if they represent something she needs to be concerned about.*

It is self-evident that we physically change as we age: all one has to do, for example, is compare the difference in the appearance of the skin between someone who is 30 years of age and someone who is 80 years of age. Differences in skin appearance may be the most obvious example of physical change with normal aging, but it is far from the only one. Indeed, age-related changes normally occur in every organ system. Table 6.1 summarizes some of these expected changes.

A frequently encountered question when caring for elderly patients is whether a given finding is normal (i.e., physiologic or generally expected for a person of that age) or abnormal (i.e., pathologic or indicative of a disease state). Distinguishing between what is physiologic and what is pathologic in a geriatric patient can be a true challenge, even for experienced clinicians.

**TABLE 6.1  Common Age-Related Changes in the Elderly**

| Organ System | Common Age-Related Changes |
| --- | --- |
| Skin | Thinning, wrinkling |
| Eyes | Cataract formation |
| Ears | Decreased hearing |
| Lungs | Decreased elasticity |
| Heart | Impaired filling |
| Arteries | Increased stiffness of arterial wall |
| Kidneys | Decreased concentrating ability |
| Muscles | Decreased muscle mass |
| Bones and joints | "Wear-and-tear" arthritic changes, decreased bone density (especially in women) |

A helpful rule-of-thumb is that a finding should be considered pathologic if it is causing bothersome symptoms. Cataracts provide a useful example. A cataract is a clouding of the lens of the eye and is thought to be related to cumulative ultraviolet light exposure. Some degree of cataract formation is a common finding in the elderly, occurring in approximately 14% of persons 65–74 years of age and approximately 32% of persons over 75 years of age (Klein, Klein, & Linton, 1992). If the cataract is mild and not causing bothersome symptoms, then surgical treatment is usually not recommended. Instead, the patient is instructed to follow up periodically with an eye doctor and also report any visual symptoms that might develop. Once bothersome symptoms arise, however, the situation changes, especially if the symptoms are adversely affecting the patient's overall level of functioning. At that point, it become slightly appropriate to propose and discuss surgical treatment so the "cataract problem" can be corrected.

Sometimes, however, a finding may be considered pathologic even in the absence of symptoms. Osteopenia (which, in its advanced form, is called osteoporosis) is frequently found in elderly patients who have no bone complaints. However, osteopenia is not an insignificant issue, even when the patient is symptom free. For example, should a woman with advanced osteopenia fall, she is clearly at higher risk of sustaining a spine or hip fracture than a person without osteopenia. Thus, to decrease their risk of fracture, women with advanced osteopenia are generally advised to follow a regimen designed to prevent further bone loss and ideally even increase the degree of bone density (Cummings et al., 1998).

In short, perhaps a more practical way for a clinician to approach the physiologic versus pathologic conundrum is to ask herself the following questions: Does anything need to be done for the patient, either measures to relieve current symptoms (or improve the patient's current level of functioning) or measures to prevent symptoms/disability from developing in the future? In essence, does the finding represent a problem that needs to be addressed?

When considering Ms. Adams' questions, therefore, how should Dr. Baker respond?

*With regard to the "wear-and-tear" arthritis, Dr. Baker informs Ms. Adams that this is a common finding in people her age. Although Ms. Adams will need medication over the next several days to control the fall-related pain (which is most likely due to a muscle/ligament contusion or "bruise"), at the present time she does not need specific medication for the arthritis because, up to this point at least, it has not been causing her any symptoms. In addition, there is no established role for preventive medication here, nor is there currently any medication that has been persuasively shown to halt or slow the progression of this type of arthritis. However, if arthritis-related symptoms develop in the future, Ms. Adams should let Dr. Baker know, as medication or other treatment interventions could certainly be offered at that time. In addition, if a medication does become available in the future that can safely and effectively prevent "back arthritis" from progressing, Dr. Baker will be sure to let Ms. Adams know.*

*With regard to the osteopenia, even though there is no fracture at the current time and even though the osteopenia has not been causing her symptoms, further interventions are indeed advisable. Dr. Baker arranges for Ms. Adams to have a bone mineral density (BMD) study, a test that provides a more accurate assessment of the degree of osteopenia. The BMD study indicates that Ms. Adams' osteopenia is relatively advanced. She is subsequently placed on a regimen designed to decrease her bone loss and, it is hoped, increase her bone density. This regimen includes an exercise program and vitamin and calcium supplementation, as well as other, more specific medication.*

## COMMON MEDICAL PROBLEMS IN THE ELDERLY

### Case 2

*Mr. Chen is an 80-year-old retired commercial artist who is accompanied by his wife for a routine follow-up visit to his physician, Dr. Dominguez.*

*Mr. Chen's list of diagnoses includes hypertension (high blood pressure); coronary artery disease, with a myocardial infarction (heart attack) four years previously; congestive heart failure secondary to systolic dysfunction (decreased pumping action of the heart); osteoarthritis (affecting both knees); and benign prostatic hypertrophy (age-related enlargement of the prostate gland, usually abbreviated as BPH). He takes nine prescribed medications, four of which he takes more than once a day. He also uses an over-the-counter antihistamine for sleep, although this is something he has never mentioned to Dr. Dominguez.*

*Mr. Chen reports he is feeling "about the same." His wife, however, expresses a number of concerns to Dr. Dominguez, including her husband's increasing forgetfulness and his two recent falls. She also indicates that coming up with funds for his multiple medications has become progressively more difficult.*

In several respects, Mr. Chen's case history is representative of the situation faced by many elderly patients.

## Multiple Chronic Medical Conditions

The elderly often suffer from multiple chronic medical conditions. For example, approximately 30% of persons 80–84 years of age have four or more chronic medical conditions (Wolff, Starfield, & Anderson, 2002). Table 6.2 lists the approximate percentage of elderly persons in the U.S. who share Mr. Chen's various medical conditions.

## Multiple Medications

The use of multiple medications is called "polypharmacy," and is a major issue confronting many elderly patients, their family caregivers,

**TABLE 6.2   Chronic Conditions in the Elderly**

| Condition | Approximate Percentage of Elderly with Condition |
| --- | --- |
| Hypertension | 50–60% (Hajjar & Kotchen, 2003) |
| Coronary artery disease (symptomatic) | 20–30% (Tresch & Aronow, 1996) |
| Congestive heart failure | 4–5% (Schocken et al., 1992) |
| Osteoarthritis (symptomatic) | 40–60% (Reginster, 2002) |
| Benign prostatic hypertrophy (symptomatic) | 30% (of men) (Chute et al., 1993) |

and their physicians. Approximately 20% of community-dwelling elders 65 years of age or older use five or more prescribed drugs per day, and that percentage is even higher when over-the-counter products are included (Kaufman et al., 2002). Polypharmacy can dramatically increase the risk of medication side effects as well as drug–drug interactions. In addition, it can impose a considerable financial burden on elderly patients and their families.

## Mental Status Changes

Mental status changes in the elderly are usually grouped into three major categories: delirium, dementia, and mild cognitive impairment (MCI). Delirium is an acute confusional state, and is commonly due either to medication or concurrent medical illness (including infections or metabolic abnormalities). Dementia is a much more chronic condition, slowly progressive over months to years, with common causes including Alzheimer's disease (50–75% of cases) and multiple strokes. MCI is a newer term, and refers to a level of cognitive impairment (including memory loss) that is less pronounced than that seen in Alzheimer's disease or other forms of dementia. To complicate matters further, it is not at all unusual for patients to have acute delirium superimposed on dementia or MCI (Fick, Agostini, & Inouye, 2002).

The prevalence of dementia rises with the age of the patient. Alzheimer's disease, for example, affects approximately 8% of persons 65 years or older and upwards of 30% of persons over age 85 years (Richards & Hendrie, 1999). The exact prevalence of MCI is unknown, but it is felt to be common and associated with significant morbidity in the elderly population (Bennett et al., 2002). Most studies looking at the prevalence of delirium have been conducted in hospitalized elders, and show that delirium affects as many as 50% of this patient population (Rummans et al., 1995).

## Falls

Falls are another common affliction of the elderly, occurring in approximately 30–60% of community-dwelling older adults each year. Falls are even more common in the elderly residents of nursing homes, with an annual incidence of approximately 1.6 falls per bed (Rubenstein & Josephson, 2002).

Falls in the elderly are usually multifactorial; that is, they typically occur because of an unfortunate combination of several factors, including physical illness, medication use, environmental hazards, and age-related impairment in balance.

## Financial Concerns

In 1998, the average expenditure for prescription drugs for an elderly person was approximately $1100 (Steinberg et al., 2000). Elders who have multiple medical conditions can have yearly medication expenditures far exceeding this national average.

What actions should Dr. Dominguez take at this point?

*Dr. Dominguez has Mr. Chen and his wife bring in all his medications from their bathroom medicine cabinet. After reviewing everything that Mr. Chen is taking, Dr. Dominquez advises discontinuation of one of the blood pressure medications, which he believes can be safely stopped at this point. Dr. Dominguez also advises Mr. Chen to stop taking the nightly over-the-counter antihistamine because such medication can be associated with falls, mental status changes, and worsening BPH (urinary) symptoms.*

*Dr. Dominquez arranges for a physical therapist to visit Mr. Chen's home to assess the home environment for fall-risk. The physical therapist offers a number of helpful recommendations, including the removal of clutter from the bedroom floor and the installation of bars along a section of the bathroom wall adjacent to the bathtub. The physical therapist also assesses Mr. Chen's gait, and determines that he would benefit from a cane.*

*Finally, Dr. Dominguez contacts a social worker to discuss Mr. Chen's financial difficulties, especially as they relate to paying for his multiple medications. The social worker discovers that Mr. Chen is eligible to receive three of his medications at a marked discount under an indigent care program recently implemented by the manufacturer.*

## DIAGNOSTIC CHALLENGES IN THE ELDERLY (INCLUDING ATYPICAL PRESENTATION OF DISEASE)

### Case 3

*Ms. Edwards, a 68-year-old saleswoman, presents to her physician, Dr. Farmer, because of a one-week history of a right-sided headache. In addition, she has noted tenderness of her scalp in the region between her right eye*

*and right ear. Ms. Edwards denies a history of similar symptoms in the
past. After further evaluation, Dr. Farmer diagnoses Ms. Edwards as
having temporal arteritis (a potentially serious inflammation of the artery
in that particular region of the scalp), a condition that is almost never
seen in people under 55 years of age.*

### Case 4

*Mr. Gordon, a retired 82-year-old machinist, is brought in by his daughter
to see their physician, Dr. Hawkins, because of a four-day history of "just
not feeling right." On further questioning of both Mr. Gordon and his
daughter, Dr. Hawkins discovers that Mr. Gordon's recent symptoms include tiredness, weakness, decreased appetite, and a mild cough not associated with sputum (phlegm), fever, chills, or shortness of breath. Mr.
Gordon's daughter also reports that her father fell in the bathroom last
night and that he seemed "a little confused" this morning. After further
evaluation, Dr. Hawkin determines that Mr. Gordon is suffering from
pneumonia. His daughter is delighted that the cause of her father's problem
has been discovered, although she is surprised that he could have pneumonia without fever, chills, or a more severe cough.*

### Case 5

*Ms. Ives, an 87-year-old great-grandmother, sees her physician, Dr. Jackson,
because of a three-day history of shortness of breath not associated with
cough, sputum, fever, chills, or chest pain. When asked why she didn't
contact Dr. Jackson when she first noticed the shortness of breath, Ms. Ives
replies that she "thought it would go away on its own" and that she "didn't
want to bother the doctors when you're all so busy." Further evaluation
reveals that Ms. Ives has suffered a recent myocardial infarction (heart
attack). She expresses disbelief when informed of the diagnosis because she
thought a "heart attack always causes chest pain."*

These three cases illustrate a number of the diagnostic challenges encountered when caring for elderly patients.

## DISEASES SPECIFIC TO THE ELDERLY

Certain diseases occur only (or almost exclusively) in the elderly. In
Case 3, Dr. Farmer needed to consider temporal arteritis as a possible

cause of Ms. Edwards' headaches, whereas that would not have been a realistic possibility in a younger patient.

## Atypical Presentation of Disease in the Elderly

For a variety of reasons (some not fully understood), disease often presents atypically in the elderly. For example, approximately 30% of patients over 80 years of age with pneumonia do not present with fever (Fernandez-Sahe et al., 2003). Similarly, elderly patients with an acute myocardial infarction often do not experience chest pain (Tresch, 1998). Other conditions, including peptic ulcer disease (Kemppainen, Raiha, & Sourander, 1997), appendicitis (Storm-Dickerson & Horattas, 2003), hyperthyroidism (Gambert, 1995), and depression (Martin, Fleming, & Evans, 1995), also commonly present atypically in the elderly.

## Non-specific Presentation of Disease:
## The Four "Common Pathways"

When the elderly are ill, they often present with non-specific complaints that don't point to a specific disease process or even a specific organ system. Instead, the presenting symptom reflects an alteration in the patient's level of functioning. The four "common pathways" of disease presentation in the elderly are:

1. Alterations in mental status: that is, acute confusion (delirium)
2. Alteration in mobility: that is, falls or other difficulties with gait (walking)
3. Alterations in continence: that is, incontinence
4. "Failure to thrive": that is, decreased appetite or non-specific tiredness or generalized weakness

In essence, when an elderly patient presents with any of the above symptoms, the physician needs to think very broadly ("casting a wide net" is the phrase clinicians often use). Possible etiologies (causes) for any of the four common pathway presentations include a variety of illnesses (including infections, myocardial infarction, stroke, metabolic abnormalities, etc.) and any one of a number of medications (both prescribed and over-the-counter). Even depression in the elderly can present in such a non-specific manner, either with mental status changes or a failure to thrive.

## Delay in Seeking Medical Care

It is common for the elderly to delay seeking medical care for the symptoms they are experiencing (Storm-Dickerson & Horattas, 2003; Tresch, Brady, Aufderheide, et al., 1996). There is good deal of speculation as to why this occurs, with several postulated explanations. Some elderly persons may assume that the symptom in question is "just due to old age" and doesn't represent an actual disease state. Other elders may be reluctant to report symptoms because they are fearful of the consequences (yet another expensive prescription, hospitalization, loss of independence, etc.). Still other elderly patients may have an underlying dementia that makes it difficult for them to express symptoms or make rational decisions about their care.

## Approach to the Elderly Patient

### Case 6

Mr. Khoury, a 66-year-old retired businessman, comes to see his new physician, Dr. Landsman, for an initial visit. Mr. Khoury has a history of adult-onset diabetes mellitus, hypothyroidism (low functioning of the thyroid gland), and gout (a type of arthritis). He is a non-smoker and he uses alcohol in moderation. He takes four prescribed medications on a regular basis as well as a daily aspirin tablet for heart protection and a daily vitamin pill. His only current symptom is a gradual worsening in his hearing. He is feeling quite well otherwise; he reports that he and his wife walk for 40 minutes five days a week and that they have an active social calendar, including helping out at a local homeless shelter for several hours each week.

Mr. Khoury has two specific questions for Dr. Landsman at today's visit: First, he wants to know what he can do "to stay as healthy as possible for as long as possible." Second, he's wondering if "now is a good time to discuss a living will" with his physician.

### Case 7

Ms. Moore is an 84-year-old retired architect who comes to see her primary care physician, Dr. Norris, for a follow-up visit. Ms. Moore is accompanied by her son and two daughters.

> *Ms. Moore has a history of metastatic breast cancer, which unfortunately has been progressing despite a recent course of chemotherapy administered by her oncologist (cancer specialist). There is currently evidence of spread of the cancer to her lungs and her bones, and she has been experiencing increasing shortness of breath as well as bone pain, the latter now unresponsive to over-the-counter pain medication. She has also been feeling progressively weaker and (in what was a very difficult decision for her) she recently decided to give up driving.*
>
> *Ms. Moore and her family have questions about what can be done for her at this stage of her illness. They are realistic about her prognosis, but want to make sure that "she is made as comfortable as possible."*

These two cases illustrate the two extremes of geriatric practice. Mr. Khoury (Case 6) is quite active and is functioning at a high level despite the presence of several chronic medical conditions. Ms. Moore (Case 7), on the other hand, has a terminal illness that will likely end her life in a matter of months. Several principles of geriatric medicine become evident as their respective physicians develop an individualized plan of care for each of them.

### Assess Patient's Functional Status

An attempt should be made to assess the functional status of each elderly patient. Table 6.3 lists "activities of daily living" (ADLs) and Table 6.4 outlines "instrumental activities of daily living" (IADLs), two tools which are commonly used to assess the functional status of elderly individuals.

Mr. Khoury probably has no deficits in any of these areas, whereas Ms. Moore is undoubtedly encountering problems with at least several IADLs, with the expectation that she will experience difficulties with at least some ADLs as her condition worsens.

**TABLE 6.3   Activities of Daily Living (ADLs)**

| Activities of Daily Living (ADLs) | |
| --- | --- |
| Bathing | Dressing |
| Grooming | Feeding |
| Toileting/continence | Transferring (e.g., from chair to bed) |

**TABLE 6.4   Instrumental Activities of Daily Living (IADLs)**

Instrumental Activities of Daily Living (IADLs)

| | |
|---|---|
| Housekeeping | Use of telephone |
| Meal preparation | Driving (or using pubic transport) |
| Shopping | Personal finances |
| Taking medications properly | |

## Maintain (and, if Possible, Improve) Patient's Functional Status

*As is obvious from his case history, Mr. Khoury is already functioning at a high level. However, Dr. Landsman has heard something in Mr. Khoury's history that raises a red flag, namely his subjective hearing loss. Dr. Landsman is aware that an uncorrected hearing deficit has the potential of causing a decline in the elderly person's quality of life as time goes on (Mulrow, Aguilar, Endicott, et al., 1990). Dr. Landsman thus arranges an audiogram (hearing test) for Mr. Khoury to evaluate this symptom further and determine if a hearing aid would benefit him. Dr. Landsman also encourages Mr. Khoury to continue with his regular exercise regimen as well as his frequent social interactions with others, knowing that these activities can exert positive effects on physical, cognitive, and psychological well-being.*

## Provide Preventive Care

Although the public often associates preventive care with children and younger adults, the elderly can also benefit from a well-designed preventive medicine approach. In the case of Mr. Khoury, preventive interventions that are reasonable to consider include vaccinations (e.g., flu shot every year in the fall, pneumococcal vaccine every 5–10 years, and tetanus booster every 10 years); colorectal cancer screening; a discussion of the pros and cons of prostate cancer screening (still a controversial issue at the current time); a blood pressure check every year; and an assessment for hyperlipidemia (with a fasting cholesterol and triglyceride panel). In addition, Mr. Khoury might be advised to maintain ideal weight, avoid excessive alcohol use, wear a seat belt whenever he rides in a car, protect himself from excessive sunlight exposure during his frequent walks (to decrease his risk of developing skin cancer), see a dentist on a regular basis, and see an eye doctor on a regular basis.

Although Ms. Moore's situation is quite different, a preventive approach might also prove beneficial to her. For example, as Ms. Moore becomes weaker and likely more bed-ridden, she will be at risk of developing decubitus ulcers (bedsores). Anticipating that possibility, Dr. Norris can consult with a nurse who specializes in wound care and then implement a plan that will lessen the chance of such a dreaded complication occurring.

## Discuss Advance Directives

"Advance directives" refers to the documentation of the preferred level of care (and specifically the aggressiveness of care) that individuals would like to receive either at the end of life or before that time, if they should become physically or mentally incapacitated. The two key components of advance directives are a living will, which typically states that the individual does not want to be kept alive through heroic efforts if there is no hope of a meaningful recovery, and a durable power of attorney for health care, in which the individual designates a surrogate charged with making health care decisions on his or her behalf if he or she is not capable of making such decisions alone.

The purpose of such advance directives is to make sure that health care professionals and families are aware of patients' specific preferences and desires so that their wishes may be honored. In many respects, the question is how best to strike a balance between quantity of life and quality of life, a balance that may well differ even among individuals within the same family. Ideally, the issue of advance directives should be discussed with elderly patients (in fact, discussed with all adult patients, elderly or not) well before a medical crisis occurs. It is thus very appropriate for Dr. Landsman to explore this topic with Mr. Khoury at the time of the initial visit, while Mr. Khoury's health is still excellent. In the case of Ms. Moore, Dr. Norris knows it is imperative at this point in her illness to have an honest, thorough, and sensitive discussion about advance directives with her and her family. Even if this issue was raised by the oncologist in the past, it would be important to review what was discussed at that time and to ask if Ms. Moore's thoughts on the matter have changed. The doctor would inquire about her understanding of her condition and her specific preferences regarding further care. To do otherwise would be to neglect an essential aspect of Ms. Moore's management in her time of greatest need (Lynn & Goldstein, 2003).

## Relieve Pain and Suffering

Relieving pain and suffering is one of the physician's primary obligations. In the case of Ms. Moore, Dr. Norris consults a palliative care team of specially trained physicians and nurses and develops a plan of care designed to relieve pain, decrease her sense of shortness of breath, prevent other symptoms from occurring (e.g., constipation, a frequent side effect of narcotic pain relievers), and provide emotional support to Ms. Moore and her family during this difficult period. Ms. Moore is enrolled in a hospice program where she receives comprehensive and compassionate care in her own home, surrounded by those she loves and those who love her. She dies peacefully in her sleep two months later, her family expressing gratitude for the humane care she received during the last several weeks of her life.

## Involve the Family

Families often provide a good deal of the care that elderly patients receive. In addition to supplying valuable information and perspective, family members can also help develop and carry out the plan of care. Working in partnership with families is key in all branches of medicine but is especially important in the world of geriatric practice.

## Use a Team Approach

Throughout this chapter, emphasis has been placed on the team approach to delivering geriatric care. In reality, even the most knowledgeable and experienced clinician needs the support, guidance, and consultative services provided by nurses, pharmacists, psychologists, physical therapists, occupational therapists, audiologists, and social workers, just to name a few of the many categories of health care professionals who use their training and skills to enhance the care of the elderly on a daily basis.

## CONCLUSION

Geriatric medicine is already an established and respected specialty in the pantheon of the healing arts, with a defined and growing body of knowledge and an approach to patients that emphasizes both practical problem solving and a respect for the human spirit. With the predicted "aging of America" over the next several decades, the need for health care professionals with expertise in geriatric medicine will only increase.

## REFERENCES

Bennett, D. A., Wilson, R. S., Schneider, J. A., Evans, D. A., Beckett, L. A., Aggarwal, N. T., Barnes, L. L., Fox, J. H., & Bach, J. (2002). Natural history of mild cognitive impairment in older persons. *Neurology, 59,* 198–205.

Chute, C. G., Panser, L. A., Girman, C. J., Oesterling, H. A., Guess, S. J., Jacobsen, S. J., & Leiber, M. M. (1993). The prevalence of prostatism: A population-based survey of urinary symptoms. *The Journal of Urology, 150,* 85–89.

Cummings, S. R., Black, D. M., Thompson, D. E., Applegate, W. B., Barrett-Connor, E., Musliner, T. A., Palermo, L., Prineas, R., Rubin, S. M., Scott, J. C., Vogt, T., Wallace, R., Yates, A. J., & LaCroix, A. Z. (1998). Effect of alendronate on risk of fracture in women with low bone density but without vertebral fractures: Results from the Fracture Intervention Trial. *Journal of the American Medical Association, 280,* 2077–2082.

Fernandez-Sahe, N., Carratala, J., Roson, B., Dorca, J., Verdaguer, R., Manresa, F., & Gudiol, F. (2003). Community-acquired pneumonia in very elderly patients: Causative organisms, clinical characteristics, and outcomes. *Medicine, 82,* 159–169.

Fick, D. M., Agostini, J. V., & Inouye, S. K. (2002). Delirium superimposed on dementia: A systematic review. *Journal of the American Geriatrics Society, 50,* 1723–1732.

Fowles, D., & Greenberg, S. (2001). *A profile of older Americans: 2000.* Washington, DC: U.S. Governmental Printing Office.

Gambert, S. R. (1995). Hyperthyroidism in the elderly. *Clinics in Geriatric Medicine, 11,* 181–188.

Hajjar, I., & Kotchen, T. A. (2003). Trends in prevalence, awareness, treatment, and control of hypertension in the United States, 1988–2000. *Journal of the American Medical Association, 290,* 199–206.

Kaufman, D. W., Kelly, J. P., Rosenberg, L., Anderson, T. E., & Mitchell, A. A. (2002). Recent patterns of medication use in the ambulatory adult population of the United States. *Journal of the American Medical Association, 287,* 337–344.

Kemppainen, H., Raiha, I., & Sourander, L. (1997). Clinical presentation of peptic ulcer disease in the elderly. *Gerontology, 43,* 283–288.

Klein, B. E. K., Klein, R., & Linton, K. L. P. (1992). Prevalence of age-related lens opacities in a population. *Ophthalmology, 99,* 546–552.

Lynn, J., & Goldstein, N. E. (2003). Advance care planning for fatal chronic illness: Avoiding commonplace errors and unwarranted suffering. *Annals of Internal Medicine, 138,* 812–818.

Martin, L. M., Fleming, K. C., & Evans, J. M. (1995). Recognition and management of anxiety and depression in elderly persons. *Mayo Clinic Proceedings, 70,* 999–1006.

Mulrow, C. D., Aguilar C., Endicott, J. E., Velez, R., Tuley, M. R., Charlip, W. S., & Hill, J. A. (1990). Association between hearing impairment and the quality of life of elderly individuals. *Journal of the American Geriatric Society, 38,* 45–50.

Reginster, J. Y. (2002). The prevalence and burden of arthritis. *Rheumatology, 41* (supplement 1), 3–6.

Richards, S. S., & Hendrie, H. C. (1999). Diagnosis, management, and treatment of Alzheimer's disease. *Archives of Internal Medicine, 159,* 789–798.

Rubenstein, L. Z., & Josephson, K. R. (2002). The epidemiology of falls and syncope. *Clinics in Geriatric Medicine, 18,* 141–158.

Rummans, T. A., Evans, J. M., Krahn, L. E., & Fleming, K. C. (1995). Delirium in elderly patients: Evaluation and management. *Mayo Clinic Proceedings, 70,* 989–998.

Schocken, D. D., Arrieta, M. I., Leaverton, P. E., & Ross, E. A. (1992). Prevalence and mortality rate of congestive heart failure in the United States. *Journal of the American College of Cardiology, 20,* 301–306.

Spillman, B. C., & Lubitz, J. (2000). The effect of longevity on spending for acute and long-term care. *New England Journal of Medicine, 342,* 1409–1415.

Steinberg, E. P., Gutierrez, B., Momani, A., Boscarino, J. A., Newman, P., & Deverka, P. (2000). Beyond survey data: A claims-based analysis of drug use and spending by the elderly. *Health Affairs, 19,* 198–211.

Storm-Dickerson, T. L., & Horattas, M. C. (2003). What have we learned in the past 20 years about appendicitis in the elderly? *American Journal of Surgery, 185,* 198–201.

Tresch, D. D. (1998). Management of the older patient with acute myocardial infarction: Difference in clinical presentations between older and younger patients. *Journal of the American Geriatric Society, 46,* 1157–1162.

Tresch, D. D., & Aronow, W. S. (1996). Clinical manifestations and diagnosis of coronary artery disease. *Clinics in Geriatric Medicine, 12*(1), 89–100.

Tresch, D. D., Brady, W. J., Aufderheide, T. P., Lawrence, S. W., & Williams, K. J. (1996). Comparison of elderly and younger patients with out-of-hospital chest pain. *Archives of Internal Medicine, 156,* 1089–1093.

Wolff, J. L., Starfield, B., & Anderson, G. (2002). Prevalence, expenditures, and complications of multiple chronic conditions in the elderly. *Archives of Internal Medicine, 162,* 2269–2276.

# 7

# Health Promotion in Later Life

*Colin Kopes-Kerr*

Although the theme of this chapter is the promotion of health and the prevention of disease in later life, it is also about taking personal responsibility for your health before you reach later life. The following hypothetical case will introduce this topic and set the stage for the issues that will be discussed here.

> You wake up one morning to find you are 50 years old. You feel good. You're satisfied with what you've done so far in your life, and you're looking forward to this day and to continuing the journey. You're boosted by the conscious awareness that none of the adversity that life has thrown at you so far has licked you. You're a survivor, and now you want to be more than that. When you reflect on it for a second time, you find yourself asking, "What can I do to make this not only last, but to become better as well?"

One can assume that all professionals and all health care consumers include a sense of well-being as one of their personal goals. Well-being, however, is a complex state of consciousness and is not limited merely to the dimensions of physical and mental health. However, it does assume some kind of optimization of health within a set of unique individual limitations. This chapter is about the simple things that can be done to promote health and wellness in later life. The important point is that this goal will not be achieved by accident; it requires deliberate planning and action.

Let's start with the most dramatic goal—we all want to avoid the desperation of a frightening terminal illness. The first step is clearly to take care of oneself now. We all need to educate ourselves about health and medical issues and their financial implications. Mere passive participation in the health care process affords only an illusory protection against the most common problems of aging. Control resides in the domain of the informed consumer. The consumer is the one hiring health professionals and contracting for their various diagnostic and therapeutic services. In this era of modern medical systems and technology we can certainly get what we want, but in order for it to make a positive difference we first have to know what we need.

## THE PERSONAL ROLE IN HEALTH

Taking care of oneself involves both a personal role and a professional role. Of the two, the personal role is more important. How do we define the personal role? It is who we are physically, nutritionally, professionally, socially, and spiritually.

When we think of ourselves, usually the first thing that comes to mind is that image in the mirror. Do we look like who we want to be? Is our weight where we want it, or have we given up? Are our muscles toned? Does our smile show healthy teeth and gums? Do our eyes show loving acceptance of the changes that age has brought on the outside?

## THE ROLE OF EXERCISE

Beyond appearance, we need to take responsibility for our vital signs. This means knowing our blood pressure and ensuring at the very least that the upper number (the systolic pressure) is less than 160. Our weight is the other big priority, but this is a tough one. The good news is that one of the most important factors relevant to our weight is entirely within our control—the amount of exercise we do on a regular basis. At least twenty minutes every day should be a goal. This is one important factor influencing longevity. The more we exercise, the longer and the better we can live and feel (Leveille et al., 1999).

## THE ROLE OF DIET

We are what we eat, which means that nutrition is critical. Here too we can really make a difference. The majority of the population takes less care of their diet as they get older, just when they need a good diet the most. Again, personal responsibility is necessary, as it is with other health promotion elements.

Medical professionals need to make individual assessments as to whether their patients are severely overweight or underweight. It has been established that being significantly overweight will shorten life expectancy (Allison, 1999; Calle, 1999; Mokdad, 1999; Oster et al., 1999; Wei, 1999). The basic principles of sound nutrition are very simple, included in which is the consumption of fiber. Statistical data for the United States shows that the average person consumes only about 15–20 grams of fiber daily whereas the recommended daily intake is 30–40 grams (DeBoer et al., 2003). Increasing fiber in our diet can easily be accomplished with cereal fiber, which appears to have the most benefits. Following the simple health rule of five servings of fiber every day is the accepted protocol (Mozaffarian et al., 2003). Fiber serves to lower cholesterol and cardiovascular risk (Rimm et al., 1996; Wolk et al., 1999; Mozaffarian et al., 2003; Liu et al., 1999), lower blood pressure, lower risk for stroke (Liu et al., 2000), lessen the risk of developing diabetes, and lower the level of sugar if you have diabetes (Liu et al., 2000). It has also been found to reduce the risk of certain cancers, particularly colon cancer (Bingham et al., 2003; Peters et al., 2003). In addition, enough fiber will benefit older people from a variety of nuisance conditions: less tendency to suffer from constipation, acid reflux, and hemorrhoids. Fruits, vegetables, and cereals are all excellent sources of fiber, and can be consumed almost without limit.

## Vitamins

The second basic principle of diet is to take a daily multivitamin (Feltcher & Fairfield, 2002; Willett & Stampfer, 2001). It doesn't really matter which; the local supermarket generic vitamin is likely to be fine. A very recent study by the Lewin Group suggests that, among the elderly, a daily vitamin may cut ultimate health care costs by up to $1.6 billion over a five-year period due to better immune function and lower heart disease risk (*Investors' Business Daily*, 2003). Recent surveys have shown that a majority of American adults consume diets deficient in more than one vitamin. Common deficiencies occur in vitamin D (Plotnikoff, 2003; Tangpricha, 2002), and vitamins C, $B_1$, $B_{12}$, and $B_6$ (Bianchetti, Rozzini, Carabellese, Zanetti, & Trabucchi, 1990), and these have important health consequences. Even after commercial grain products are fortified, many adults don't get enough folic acid, which appears to substantially lower the risk of vascular disease, heart attack, stroke, and even Alzheimer's disease (Rimm et al., 1998; Robinson et al., 1998); if taken for a period of 10 years or more, it can reduce the risk of colon cancer by as much as two-thirds (Feltcher & Fairfield, 2002). Vitamin $B_6$ is similarly important for preventing both heart disease and colon cancer. Multivitamins have been found to reduce the risk of cataracts (Kuzniarz, 2001). Antioxidants, namely, vitamin C, vitamin E, and beta-carotene, appear to delay progression in patients with age-related macular degeneration (*The Medical Letter*, 2003). For those undergoing cardiac interventions such as angioplasty, supplementation with folic acid, vitamin $B_{12}$, and vitamin $B_6$ (pyridoxine) has been found to dramatically reduce the risk of heart attack and death in the year after the procedure (Schnyder et al., 2001; Schnyder et al., 2002). Patients with diabetes who take a multivitamin supplement experience fewer infectious illnesses (Barringer, Kirk, Santaniella, Foley, & Michielutte, 2003). Chronic deficiency of vitamin D is one of the leading risk factors for osteoporosis and hip and wrist fractures, with all the disability, frailty, and even mortality that go along with it. The vertebral fractures associated with osteoporosis are the leading cause of low back pain as we get older. All of this can be prevented by a simple combination of exercise and supplementation with calcium and vitamin D (Trivedi, 2003). Taking extra calcium (up to 1000 mg/day) has been found to improve cholesterol levels (Reid et al., 2002), help in weight loss (Zemel et al., 2002), prevent diabetes (Pereira, Jacobs, Van Horn, Slattery, Kartashov, & Ludwig, 2002), and reduce the risk of colon cancer (Baron et al., 1999).

## Fish

The third basic principle of diet is to increase the amount of fish consumed. Fish and fish-oil (T-3 fatty acids) can significantly reduce the risk of heart disease and heart attack by up to 30% (Bucher, Hengstler, Schindler, & Meier, 2002), sudden cardiac death by up to 45% (*Prescriber's Letter*, 2002), stroke (He et al., 2002), and even possibly Alzheimer's disease (Friedland, 2003; Morris et al., 2003). At least 2 servings of fish each week is recommended.

## The Question of Fat

Although fat has received the most general public attention in diet, it is ultimately not as important as once thought. At present it is not clear which diets, low-fat or low-carbohydrate, are best for those who want to lose weight and reduce cardiovascular risk, nor is it clear what is the ideal proportion of various kinds of fats: saturated, monounsaturated, trans-saturated, and polyunsaturated. It is probably best to be less concerned about fat consumption until research produces better answers.

In general either a "prudent" or Mediterranean-style diet (high in vegetables, fruits, and grains) is more healthy than our typical high-fat, low-fiber, meat-based American diet (Bravata, 2003). The two most important dietary goals are to reduce the total number of calories consumed each day by a small amount (Bonow, 2003), and to try to modify overall diet in the direction of the Mediterranean diet. An effort should be made to bring as many of our ordinary daily food choices into conformity as possible without obsessing about them (de Lorgeril et al., 1999; Fuentes, Lopez-Miranda, Sanchez, Sanchez, Paez, & Paz-Rojas, 2001). One can evaluate one's own diet for its "Mediterranean-ness" by calculating a "Mediterranean Diet Score"; score 1 point for each of the following dietary habits: above-average consumption of vegetables, legumes, fruits, nuts, cereal, and fish; below-average consumption of meat, poultry, and dairy products; moderate alcohol intake. A recent study has shown that increasing one's Mediterranean diet score by as little as 2 points over a 3 to 4 year period is associated with up to a 33% reduction in coronary mortality, a 24% reduction in cancer, and a 25% reduction in total mortality (Trichopoulou et al., 2003).

## LIFE WORK AND ATTITUDE

Our choice of work or profession, and particularly our choice of the manner and intensity with which we pursue our profession is extremely important to overall health. We should all try to engage in work that has a high degree of meaning for us, doing what we enjoy, but at the same time, we need to slow down. It is fine to be a Type A personality, driven, multitasking and high achieving, but controls are necessary for balance. Work heals, but stress kills. The higher the intensity of one's occupation, the more one needs to establish specific, regular, formal time-outs for silence, and doing nothing. Dr. Deepak Chopra (1993) prescribes 15 minutes of silence twice a day every day. A number of studies show that regular time spent in meditation leads to significantly lower blood pressure, lessened perception of pain and stress, and reduced cardiovascular risk (Barrows & Jacobs, 2003; Hall, 2003; Kabat-Zinn, 1990; Ornish et al., 1990; Schneider, 1995; Stein, 2003). It also has been found to be directly related to increased energy, feeling more refreshed, and invigorated moment-to-moment living. Emptying our minds regularly by the practice of silence helps us to experience awe and the full dimensions of who we are; it enables us to perceive our life's meaning and purpose distinct from the noise and clutter of everyday life.

Work either outside the home or taking care of family may be our true purpose, but we might never know unless we take the time to reflect.

## SOCIAL ACTIVITY

Science has shown that human beings are intensely, and necessarily, social creatures. Creating and fostering relationships, and all the support that this implies, is known to be related to good health. Intimacy, family, partnership, collaboration, planning, and institution building are all functions of who we are with and how much we value those relationships. To form and nurture these relationships requires time, and the only way to increase time is to let go of something else. Life is about progress in letting go gracefully. If we know who we are and what we value, letting go of the little stuff is easy.

One of the interesting developments in recent gerontology research has been, not the finding of a cure for Alzheimer's disease, which is still elusive, but finding multiple ways to possibly prevent it. Fostering social networks and relationships was found to be one possible way to prevent cognitive decline (Bassuk, Glass, & Berkman, 1999). The "use it or lose it" principle can be implemented by just exercising our minds regularly in simple pursuits such as crossword puzzles, following the stock market, or computing baseball averages (Ball et al., 2002; Press & Alexander, 2003; Verghese et al., 2003; Wilson et al., 2002).

## THE MEDICAL ASPECTS OF HEALTH: GETTING THE BIG PICTURE

The steps above take care of life's basics for health—the simple, human, living non-medical aspects. From more traditional medical perspectives, recent data suggest that adopting health promotion efforts before the age of 65 affords us the opportunity to significantly improve our health and longevity without increasing future health care costs significantly (Lubitz, Cai, Kramarow, & Lentzner, 2003). There is one area of health and medical care that is more important than any of the others by far: the prevention of heart disease, which is the number one cause of adult death in the United States. The primary and most effective medical intervention is the simple coronary artery disease risk assessment. Primary care physicians should be regularly asking their patients about the eight primary cardiac risk factors: (1) age (risk increases substantially after age 50 for men and age 60 for women), (2) sex (risk increases for males), (3) family history of premature heart disease (risk increases if any first degree relative had a heart attack or coronary intervention before age 55 for men and age 65 for women), (4) high cholesterol (and related lipid substances), (5) smoking, (6) high blood pressure, (7) diabetes (having diabetes carries with it the same risk for a heart attack as having either angina or a prior heart attack), and (8) lack of regular exercise. Recent studies have justified adding a ninth risk factor to this list, which is weight. Simple obesity alone does not appear to be an independent cardiac risk factor, but if it is associated with specific abnormalities of the lipids in the blood, it is. These important lipid disturbances (beyond the distinct and separate risk related to choles-terol) are a "good cholesterol" (HDL cholesterol) level that is too low, combined with a triglyceride level that is too high, a condition known as "insulin resistance" (Reaven, 2003).

What is impressive is that just the simple process of reviewing this global cardiac risk assessment itself leads to lower risks apparently by the virtue of the implicit educational intervention, even before physicians undertake any specific, targeted interventions (Engberg, Christensen, Karlsmose, Lous, & Lauritzen, 2002). The reason for this appears to be the power of the educational relationship between physician and pa-tient; when this is done regularly and systematically, it leads inevitably to changes in awareness that get reflected in active changes in behavior that result in better health.

There are certain factors such as sex, age, and family history that we have no control over. Genetics play a real role in health, but this can often be compensated for by the control we do have over other things. If we focus on exercise, for example, there is reason to believe that even with a family history of heart disease, we can still lower our cardiac risk. If we add proper nutrition awareness and behaviors (multivitamin supplements, folic acid, and increased fiber, for example), we can fur-ther lower risk. For those with specific risk factors to begin with, such as high cholesterol, working with a health care professional and taking medication offer additional major gains.

For those who want to measure these risks in terms of real numbers, modern science and Internet technology make it easy. There are simple computer calculators available on the Internet to allow people to enter these numbers for themselves and calculate their health risks. Based on large-scale data from the Framingham population studies, which consisted mostly of middle-aged white adults, we can calculate our numerical probability of having a heart attack, given our current lifestyle characteristics (National Heart, Lung, and Blood Institute, 2003). There are also calculations based on diverse populations, including almost all ethnic and racial groups, which are even more accurate. This is especially important because many health providers do not take these factors into consideration. This is one of the best ways to determine whether your health provider is practicing the best medicine, if he or she is taking all of these elements into consideration.

## MORTALITY RATES AND PREMATURE DEATHS

Studying the causes of premature death is important, as we tend to run into very predictable but preventable health problems. A small number of risk factors account for the large majority of premature deaths. Data compiled by the Centers for Disease Control show that in 2002, five problems accounted for 68% of all deaths: heart disease (29%), cancer (23%), stroke (7%), chronic lung disease (5%), and motor vehicle accidents (4%). The other causes of death in order of prevalence are diabetes (3%), pneumonia and influenza (3%), Alzheimer's disease (<2%), renal disease and kidney failure (<2%), sepsis (bacterial invasion of the blood stream) (<2%), suicide (<2%), chronic liver disease and cirrhosis (<2%), hypertension-related renal disease (<2%), homicide (<2%), and pneumonia due to accidental ingestion of oral or stomach contents into the lungs (<2%) (Centers for Disease Control, 2004). These numbers suggest concentrating on improving only several health habits can result in large dividends in health and longevity.

## KEEPING HEALTHY: THE CORE HABITS

As we get older we become more prone to the major health risks mentioned above. However, individuals still retain a lot of control over their health. Never underestimate the profound effects of these simple habits including:

- Eating 3 balanced meals a day with 5 servings of fruits and vegetables, regular fish, and a daily multivitamin with folic acid (Fung et al., 2003; Giovannucci et al., 1995; Joshipura et al., 1999; Leiberman et al., 2003; Rohan et al., 2000)
- Exercising, even just a daily brisk 20-minute walk (Blumenthal et al., 1999; Manson et al., 1992; Toumilehto et al., 2001; Waldholz, 2003)
- Avoiding tobacco products, excess alcohol, recreational drugs, and excessive use of prescription medications

- Taking an aspirin or a baby aspirin every day, under medical supervision (Baron et al., 2003; Hayden et al., 2002; Sandler et al., 2003)
- Partnering with a health professional to plan and follow a healthy lifestyle (Josefson, 2003; Knowler et al., 2002)

On a regular basis, as adults grow older, they should:

- Assess their specific Coronary Artery Disease Risk Score and review all 9 factors, deciding where personal risk factors exist, and making a plan for what to do about elevated blood pressure and cholesterol.
- Check blood pressure and keep it under control.
- Make sure immunizations are adequate and up-to-date. All adults over 50 should receive influenza vaccine and, at age 55, immunization against systemic disease from the pneumonia germ (*Pneumovax*). All adults should also be sure their tetanus immunization has been boosted within the last 10 years.
- Review medications for potential side effects and eliminate any that are not absolutely necessary.
- Have a frank talk with their health provider about the various cancer risks. Determine which are most relevant, and which offer a balance of risk vs. benefits that is personally compelling. Included should be annual breast screening, Pap smears, and mammograms for women, and prostate cancer screening for men. Colon cancer screening should be discussed for all adults over 50 years of age.
- Make a plan for which periodic or annual blood tests are necessary. Recommended are checking cholesterol, possibly a full lipid panel, kidney function, glucose (sugar), and the protein screening test for diabetes, blood count (to identify anemia), liver function tests if taking certain medications known to affect the liver, and potassium or other mineral levels if they are on certain other medications, and a periodic thyroid function test.

Staying healthy is neither mysterious or difficult. It merely takes a decision to do it. This is not to say that we can all avoid all of the hazards of life, disease, and aging. What we can do is to optimize the status of our bodies and the state of our minds, over which we do have some control.

## PROPOSED PHARMACOLOGICAL THERAPY

It has been recently proposed that some pharmacological therapies, simple medications that may promote wellness and prevent illness, may help assure a long and healthy life. With proper medical supervision, these are neither complicated nor risky. One such therapy has been suggested by Wald and Law (2003), known as the "Polypill Report." This analysis suggests that if individuals who reached the age of 55 started taking one pill a day, they could reduce the risk of heart disease by 88% and the risk of stroke by 80%. The hypothetical "Polypill," as its name suggests, is a combination of ingredients, all of which have well-established track records of safety and efficacy, but none-the-less require medical supervision. Most of the six proposed ingredients of this pill should be familiar: aspirin (one baby tablet), folic acid (800 micrograms), a cholesterol-lowering medication (either simvastatin, (Zocor) 40 mg, or atorvastatin (Lipitor), 10 mg, and a half-dose of the three most effective blood-pressure lowering agents: hydrochlorothiazide (a diuretic), enalapril (an ACE-inhibitor), and atenolol (a beta-blocker). The estimated magnitude of the benefit of these common and inexpensive medications has been found to be astounding (Wald & Law, 2003). The philosophy of such an intervention is fully consistent with the basic approach and emphasis outlined in this chapter. Add to this a few modest but sound dietary changes, a multivitamin and minerals, exercise and meditation, and older adults are well on their way to the long and happy life they desire. However, adding the above medications in otherwise well individuals should be discussed with their physicians.

## CONCLUSION

No one has more power or control over our health than we do. No one can do a better job of taking care of us than we can, if we make a habit of knowing ourselves, knowing our bodies, and reflecting on our choices. The message is inevitably and reassuringly redundant: there are just a few things that we need to do, fostering a few basic good habits such as eating right, exercising, directly assessing cardiac risk, modifying any cardiac risk factors to the extent that we can, and avoiding toxic substances like tobacco and second-hand smoke and excess alcohol. When we add other positive health habits such as regular immunizations and adhering to basic safety practices, it will undoubtedly result in the promotion of health and the prevention of disease.

## REFERENCES

Allison, D. B., Fontaine, K. R., Manson, J. E., Stevens, J., & VanItallie, T. B. (1999). Annual deaths attributable to obesity in the U.S. *Journal of the American Medical Association, 282,* 1530–1538.

Ball, K., Berch, D. B., Helmers, K. F., Jobe, J. B., Leveck, M. D., Marsiske, M., Morris, J. N., Rebok, G. W., Smith, D. M., & Willis, S. L. (2002). Effects of cognitive training interventions with older adults: A randomized controlled trial. *Journal of the American Medical Association, 288*(18), 2271–2281.

Baron, J. A., Beach, M., Mandel, J. S., van Stolk, R. U., Haile, R. W., Sandler, R. S., Rothstein, R., Summers, R. W., Snover, D. C., Beck, G. J., Bond, J. H., & Greenberg, E. R. (1999). Calcium supplements for the prevention of colorectal adenomas. *The New England Journal of Medicine, 340,* 101–107.

Baron, J. A., Cole, B. F., Sandler, R. S., Haile, R. W., Ahnen, D., Braselier, R., Summers, R. W., Rothstein, R., Burke, C. A., Shover, D. C., Church, T. R., Allen, J. I., Beach, W., Beck, G. J., Bond, J. H., Byers, T., Greenberg, E. R., Mandel, J. S., Marcon, N., Pearson, L., Saibil, F., & Stolk, R. U. (2003). A randomized trial of aspirin to prevent colorectal adenomas. *The New England Journal of Medicine, 348*(89), 1–9.

Barringer, T. A., Kirk, J. K., Santaniello, A. C., Foley, K. L., & Michielutte, R. (2003). Effect of a multivitamin and mineral supplement on infection and quality of life: A randomized, double-blind, placebo-controlled trial. *Annals of Internal Medicine, 138,* 365–371.

Barrows, K. A., & Jacobs, B. P. (2003). Mind–body medicine: An introduction and review of the literature. *Complementary and Alternative Medicine, 86*(1), 11–31.

Bassuk, S. S., Glass, T. A., & Berkman, L. F. (1999). Social disengagement and incident cognitive decline in community-dwelling elderly persons. *Annals of Internal Medicine, 131,* 165–173.

Bianchetti, A., Rozzini, R., Carabellese, C., Zanetti, O., & Trabucchi, M. (1990). Nutritional intake, socioeconomic conditions, and health status in a large elderly population. *Journal of the American Geriatrics Society, 38,* 521–526.

Bingham, S. A., Day, N. E., Luben, R., Ferrari, P., Slimani, N., Norat, T., Clavel-Chapelon, F., Kesse, E., Nieters, A., Boeing, H., Tjonneland, A., Overvad, K., & Martinez, C. (2003). Dietary fiber in food and protection against colorectal cancer in the European Prospective Investigation into Cancer and Nutrition (EPIC): An observational study. *Lancet, 361,* 1496–1501.

Blumenthal, J. A., Babyak, M. A., Moore, K. A., Craighead, W. E., Herman, S., Knatri, P., Waugh, R., Napolitano, M. A., Forman, L. M., Appelbaum, M., & Doraiswamy, P. M. (1999). Effects of exercise training on older patients with major depression. *Archives of Internal Medicine, 159,* 2349–2356.

Bonow, R. O., & Eckel, R. H. (2003). Diet, obesity and cardiovascular risk. *New England Journal of Medicine, 348*(21), 2057–2058.

Bravata, D. M., Sanders, L., Huang, J., Krumholz, H. M., Olkin, I., & Gardner, C. D. (2003). Efficacy and safety of low-carbohydrate diets: A systematic review. *Journal of the American Medical Association, 289*(14), 1837–1850.

Bucher, H. C., Hengstler, P., Schindler, C., & Meier, G. (2002). N–3 polyunsaturated fatty acids in coronary heart disease: A meta-analysis of randomized controlled trials. *American Journal of Medicine, 112,* 298–304.

Calle, E. E., Thun, M. J., Petrelli, J. M., Rodriguez, C., & Heath, C. Jr. (1999). Body-mass index and mortality in a prospective cohort of U.S. adults. *New England Journal of Medicine, 341,* 1097–1105.

Centers for Disease Control. (2004). The National Center for Injury Prevention and Control: WISQARS: Leading Causes of Death Reports. "Data from 1999 and later." Available at: http://webappa.cdc.gov/sasweb/ncipc/leadcaus.html; accessed June 2, 2004.

Chopra, D. (1993). *Ageless body, timeless mind: The quantum alternative to growing old.* New York: Harmony Books.

DeBoer, S. W., Thomas, R. J., Brekke, M. J., Brekke, L. N., Hoffman, R. S., Menzel, P. A., Aase, L. A., Hayes, S. N., & Kottke, T. E. (2003). Dietary intake of fruits, vegetables, and fat in Olmsted County, Minn. *Mayo Clinic Proceedings, 78,* 161–166.

de Lorgeril, M., Salen, P., Martin, J., Monjaud, I., Delaye, J., & Mamelle, N. (1999). Mediterranean diet, traditional risk factors, and the rate of cardiovascular complications after myocardial infarction: Final report of the Lyon Diet Heart Study. *Circulation, 99,* 779–785.

Engberg, M., Christensen, B., Karlsmose, B., Lous, J., & Lauritzen, T. (2002). General health screenings to improve cardiovascular risk profiles: A randomized controlled trial in general practice with 5-year follow-up. *Journal of Family Practice, 51*(6), 546–552.

Feltcher, R. H., & Fairfield, K. M. (2002). Vitamins for chronic disease prevention in adults: Clinical applications. *Journal of the American Medical Association, 287,* 3127–3129.

Friedland, R. P. (2003). Fish consumption and the risk of Alzheimer Disease: Is it time to make dietary recommendations? (Editorial) *Archives of Neurology, 60,* 923–924.

Fuentes, F., Lopez-Miranda, J., Sanchez, E., Sanchez, F., Paez, J., & Paz-Rojas, E. (2001). Mediterranean and low-fat diets improve endothelial function in hypercholesterolemic men. *Annals of Internal Medicine, 134,* 1115–1119.

Fung, T., Hu, F. B., Fuchs, C., Giovannucci, E., Hunter, D. J., Stampfer, M. J., Colditz, G. A., & Willett, W. C. (2003). Major dietary patterns and the risk of colorectal cancer in women. *Archives of Internal Medicine, 163,* 309–314.

Giovannucci, E., Rimm, E. B., Ascherio, A., Stampfer, M. J., Colditz, G. A., & Willett, W. C. (1995). Alcohol, low-methionine-low-folate diets, and risk of colon cancer in men. *Journal of the National Cancer Institute, 87,* 265–273.

Hall, S. S. (2003, September 14). Is Buddhism good for your health? *The New York Times Magazine,* pp. 46–49.

Hayden, M., Pignone, M., Phillips, C., & Mulrow, C. (2002). Aspirin for the primary prevention of cardiovascular events: A summary of the evidence for the U.S. Preventive Services Task Force. *Annals of Internal Medicine, 136,* 161–172.

He, K., Rimm, E. B., Merchant, A., Rosner, B. A., Stampfer, M. J., Colditz, G. A., & Willett, W. C. (2002). Fish consumption and risk of stroke in men. *Journal of the American Medical Association, 288,* 3130–3136.

*Investors' Business Daily.* (2003, October 3). Trends & Innovations. Vitamins can cut health care costs, p. A2.

Josefson, D. (2003). Statins may reduce risk of depression. *British Medical Journal, 327,* 467. citing Young-Xu, Y., Blatt, B. C., Chan, K. A., Liao, J. K., Ravid, S., & Blatt, C. M. (2001). Long-term statin use and psychological well-being. *Journal of the American College of Cardiology, 42,* 690–697.

Joshipura, K. J., Ascherio, A., Manson, J. E., Stampfer, M. J., Rimm, E. B., Spiezer, F. E., Hennekens, C. H., Spiegelman, D., & Willett, W. C. (1999). Fruit and vegetable intake in relation to risk of ischemic stroke. *Journal of the American Medical Association, 283,* 1233–1239.

Kabat-Zinn, J. (1990). Full catastrophe living: Using the wisdom of your body and mind to face stress, pain, and illness. *Delta, 45,* 19–20.

Knowler, W. C., Barrett-Connor, E., Fowler, S. E., Hamman, R. F., Lachin, J. M., Walker, E. A., & Nathan, D. M. (2002). Reduction in the incidence of type 2 diabetes with lifestyle intervention or metformin. *New England Journal of Medicine, 346,* 393–403.

Kuzniarz, M. (2001). The use of vitamin supplements and cataract: The Blue Mountains Eye Study. *American Journal of Ophthalmology, 132,* 19–26.

Leveille, S. G., Guralnik, J. M., Ferrucci, L., & Langlois, J. A. (1999). Aging successfully until death in old age: Opportunities for increased active life expectancy. *American Journal of Epidemiology, 149,* 654–664.

Lieberman, D. A., Prindiville, S., Weiss, D. G., & Willett, W. for the VA Cooperative Study Group. (2003). Risk factors for advanced colonic neooplasia and hyperplastic polyps in asymptomatic individuals. *Journal of the American Medical Association, 290,* 2959–2967.

Liu, S., Manson, J. E., Stampfer, M. J., Rexrode, K. M., Hu, F. B., Rimm, E., & Willett, W. C. (2000). Whole grain consumption and risk of ischemic stroke in women: A prospective study. *Journal of the American Medical Association, 284,* 1534–1540.

Liu, S., Stampfer, M. J., Hu, F. B., Giovannucci, E., Rimm, E., Manson, J. E., Hennekens, C. H., & Willett, W. C. (1999). Whole grain consumption and risk of coronary heart disease: Results from the Nurses' Health Study. *American Journal of Clinical Nutrition, 70,* 412–419.

Lubitz, J., Cai, L., Kramarow, E., & Lentzner, H. (2003). Life expectancy and health care spending among the elderly. *New England Journal of Medicine, 349,* 1048–1055.

Manson, J. E., Nathan, D. M., Krolewski, A. S., Stampfer, M. J., Willett, W. C., & Hennekens, C. H. (1992). A prospective study of exercise and incidence of diabetes among U.S. male physicians. *Journal of the American Medical Association, 268,* 63–67.

Mokdad, A. H., Serdula, M. K., Dietz, W. H., Bowmn, B. A., Marks, J. S., & Koplan, J. P. (1999). The spread of the obesity epidemic 1991–1998. *Journal of the American Medical Association.*

Morris, M. C., Evans, D. A., Bienias, J. L., Tangney, C. C., Bennett, D. A., Wilson, R. S., Aggarwal, N., & Schneider, J. (2003). Consumption of fish and −3 fatty acids and risk of incident Alzheimer Disease. *Archives of Neurology, 60,* 940–946.

Mozaffarian, D., Kumanyika, S. K., Lemaitre, R. N., Olson, J. L., Burke, G. L., & Siscovic, D. S. (2003). Cereal, fruit, and vegetable fiber intake and the risk of cardiovascular disease in elderly individuals. *Journal of the American Medical Association, 289,* 1659–1666.

National Heart, Lung, and Blood Institute (NHLBI). (2003, November). Web-based calculator. Available at http://hin.nhlbi.nih.gov/atpiii/calculator.asp

Ornish, D., Brown, S., Scherwitz, L., Billings, J. H., Armstrong, W. T., Ports, T. A., McLanahan, S. M., Kirkeede, R. L., Brand, R. J., & Gould, K. L. (1990). Can lifestyle changes reverse coronary heart disease?: The Lifestyle Heart Trial. *Lancet, 336,* 129–133.

Oster, G., Thompson, D., Edelsberg, J., Bird, A. P., & Colditz, G. A. (1999). Lifetime health and economic benefits of weight loss among obese persons. *American Journal of Public Health, 789,* 1536–1542.

Pereira, M. A., Jacobs, D. R., Van Horn, L., Slattery, M. L., Kartashov, A. I., & Ludwig, D. S. (2002). Calcium consumption, obesity, and the insulin resistance syndrome in young adults: The CARDIA Study. *Journal of the American Medical Association, 287,* 2081–2089.

Peters, U., Sinha, R., Chatterjee, N., Subar, A. F., Ziegler, R. G., Kulldorf, M., Bresalier, R., Weissfield, J. L., Flood, A., Schatzkin, A., & Hayes, R. B. (2003). Dietary fiber and colorectal adenoma in a colorectal cancer early detection programme. *Lancet, 361,* 1491–1495.

Plotnikoff, G. A., & Quigley, J. M. Prevalence of severe hypovitaminosis D in patients with persistent, nonspecific musculoskeletal pain. *Mayo Clinic Proceedings 2003, 78,* 1463–1470.

Prescriber's Letter (2002). Vol 9 No 5: page 30; detail document #180510. O'Mara, N. B. Fish and fish oil and cardiovascular disease.

Press, D., & Alexander, M. (2003, October). Prevention of dementia. *UptoDate in Family Practice,* p. 3.

Reaven, G. M. (2003). Importance of identifying the overweight patients who will benefit the most by losing weight. *Annals of Internal Medicine, 138,* 420–423.

Reid, I. R., Mason, B., Horne, A., Ames, R., Clearwater, J., Brava, U., Orr-Walker, B., Wu, F., Evans, M. C., & Gamble, G. D. (2002). Effects of calcium supplementation on serum lipid concentration in normal older women: A randomized controlled trial. *American Journal of Medicine, 112,* 343–347.

Rimm, E. B., Ascherio, A., Giovannucci, E., Spiegelman, D., Stampfer, M. J., & Willett, W. C. (1996). Vegetable, fruit, and cereal fiber intake and risk of coronary heart disease among men. *Journal of the American Medical Association, 275,* 447–452.

Rimm, E. B., Willett, W. C., Hu, F. B., Sampson, L., Colditz, G. A., Manson, J. E., Hennekens, C., & Stampfer, M. J. (1998). Folate and vitamin B6 from diet and supplements in relation to risk of coronary heart disease among women. *Journal of the American Medical Association, 279,* 359–364.

Robinson, K., Arheart, K., Refsum, H., Brattstrom, L., Boers, G., Ueland, P., Rubba, P., Palma-Reis, R., Meleady, R., Daly, R., Witterman, J., & Graham, I. (1998). Low circulating folate and vitamin B6 concentrations: Risk factors for stroke, peripheral vascular disease, and coronary artery disease. *Circulation, 97,* 437–443.

Rohan, T. E., Jain, M. G., Howe, G. R., & Miller, A. B. (2000). Dietary folate consumption and breast cancer risk. *Journal of the National Cancer Institute, 92,* 266–269.

Sandler, R. S., Halabi, S., Baron, J. A., Budinger, S., & Paskett, E. (2003). A randomized trial of aspirin to prevent colorectal adenomas in patients with previous colorectal cancer. *New England Journal of Medicine, 348,* 884–890.

Schneider, R. H., Staggers, F., Alexander, C. N., Sheppard, W., Rainforth, M., & Kondwani, K. (1995). A randomized controlled trial of stress reduction for hypertension in older African Americans. *Hypertension, 26,* 280–287.

Schnyder, G., Roffi, M., Flammer, Y., Pin, R., & Hess, O. M. (2002). Effect of homocysteine-lowering therapy with folic acid, vitamin B12, and vitamin B6 on clinical outcome after percutaneous coronary intervention: The Swiss Heart Study: A randomized controlled trial. *Journal of the American Medical Association, 288,* 973–979.

Schnyder, G., Roffi, M., Pin, R., Flammer, Y., Lange, H., Eberli, F. R., Meier, B., Turi, Z. G., & Hess, O. M. (2001). Decreased rate of coronary restenosis after lowering of plasma homocysteine levels. *New England Journal of Medicine, 345,* 1593–1600.

Stein, J. (2003, August 4). Just Say "Om." *Time,* pp. 49–56.

Tangpricha, V. (2002). Vitamin D insufficiency among free-living healthy young adults. *American Journal of Medicine, 112,* 659–662.

The Medical Letter (2003). Antioxidant vitamins and zinc for macular degeneration. *The Medical Letter, 45,* No 1158: 45–46.

Trichopoulou, A., Costacou, T., Bamia, C., & Trichopoulos, D. (2003). Adherence to Mediterranean diet and survival in a Greek population. *New England Journal of Medicine, 348,* 2599–2608.

Trivedi, D. P., Doll, R., & Khaw, K. T. (2003). The effect of four monthly oral vitamin D3 (cholecalciferol) supplementation on fractures and mortality in men and women living in the community: Randomised double blind controlled trial. *British Medical Journal, 326,* 469–472.

Tuomilehto, J., Lindstrom, J., Eriksson, J. G., Valle, T. T., Hamalainen, H., Hanne-Parikka, P., Keinanen-Kinkuanniemi, S., Laakso, M., Lougheranto, A., Rastas, M., Salminen, V., & Unsitupa, M. (2001). Prevention of type 2 diabetes mellitus by changes in lifestyle among subjects with impaired glucose tolerance. *New England Journal of Medicine, 344,* 1343–1350.

Verghese, J., Lipton, R. B., Katz, M. J., Hall, C. B., Derby, C. A., Kuslansky, G., Ambrose, A. F., Sliwinski, M., & Buschke, H. (2003). Leisure activities and the risk of dementia in the elderly. *New England Journal of Medicine, 348*(2), 2508–2516.

Wald, N. J., & Law, M. R. (2003). A strategy to reduce cardiovascular disease by more than 80%. *British Medical Journal, 326,* 1419–1423.

Waldholz, M. (2003, October 24). Breast cancer & exercise: Gene mutations pose greater cancer threat, study finds. *The Wall Street Journal,* pp. B1, B2.

Wei, M., Kampert, J. B., Barlow, C. E., Nichaman, M. Z., Gibbons, L. W., Paffenbarger, R. S. Jr, & Blair, S. N. (1999). The relationship between low cardiorespiratory fitness and mortality in normal-weight, overweight, and obese men. *Journal of the American Medical Association, 282,* 1547–1553.

Willett, W. C., & Stampfer, M. J. (2001). What vitamins should I be taking, Doctor? *New England Journal of Medicine, 345*(25), 1819–1824.

Wilson, R. S., Mendes, C. F., Barnes, L. L., Schneider, J. A., Bienias, J. L., Evans, D. A., & Bennett, D. A. (2002). Participation in cognitively stimulating activities and risk of incident Alzheimer's disease. *Journal of the American Medical Association, 287,* 742–748.

Wolk, A., Manson, J. E., Stampfer, M. J., Colditz, G. A., Hu, F. B., Speizer, F. E., Hennekers, C. H., & Willett, W. C. (1999). Long term intake of dietary fiber and decreased risk of coronary heart disease among women. *Journal of the American Medical Association, 281,* 1998–2004.

Zemel, B., Thompson, W., Zemel, P., Nocton, A., Milstead, A., Morris, K., & Campbell, P. (2002). Dietary calcium and dairy products accelerate weight and fat loss during energy restriction in obese adults. *American Journal of Clinical Nutrition, 75,* 342S–343S.

# 8

# Considerations for Oral Health in the Elderly

## Brenda M. Horrell

G ood oral health contributes to success in the aging process by enhancing self-esteem, appearance, self-image, socialization, nutrition, and dietary selection (Fiske, 2000). Oral health care for the older person includes issues that are relevant to younger people as well, such as good oral hygiene and diet, preventive and restorative care, and esthetics. However there are additional issues that are specific to an older population, needs that are related to their changing health status, as well as possible changes to their care and living arrangements. The summary of the Surgeon General's Report (SGR) (2000) on oral health in America carried the major message that oral health means much more than healthy teeth and is integral to the general health and well-being of all Americans. Additionally, oral diseases and disorders affect health and well-being throughout life. Furthermore, the SGR noted that the older population is often at risk for disease and can experience limited access to oral health care due to place of residence, economic factors, social isolation, complex medical illness, and other individual and social factors (Pyle & Stoller, 2003). Specifically, the SGR highlighted the following points related to geriatric oral health care:

1. Disparities remain for access-limited groups despite oral health care improvement for many Americans.
2. Dentists have the opportunity to play an expanded role in the interdisciplinary health care team.
3. The integration of general and oral health care programs is insufficient.
4. The public health structure is not sufficient to the needs of access-limited groups.

5. Medically necessary oral health care remains limited, especially for the elderly.
6. The new dental practice choices may reflect the debt-load of the dentist at graduation.
7. Long-term care facilities have limited capacity to deliver needed oral health care services.

A coordinated effort can overcome the educational, environmental, social, health systems, and financial barriers that have created vulnerable populations whose oral health is at risk.

In order to better understand the need for greater interdisciplinary training in gerontology, one must have a better understanding of the diverse health problems, both oral and general, that are encountered in this population. Older adults comprise a diverse group in terms of age cohorts, health, income, interests, and racial and ethnic backgrounds. Additionally, the older adult population may be divided into three health categories: the healthy and well senior, the medically compromised senior, and the high health risk senior. In the United States, approximately 85% of seniors live in their community, 10% are considered homebound (disabled, but not institutionalized), and 5% reside in nursing homes or assisted living facilities (Niessen & Gibson, 2000). The variability of the attributes of this diverse population may be significant in terms of consideration of the issues that affect the process of dental treatment planning (Berg, Garcia, & Berkey, 2000).

## AGE-RELATED CHANGES TO ORAL HEALTH

It is of primary importance to differentiate between characteristics of normative aging, that is, changes related solely to the aging process that are progressive, universal, and non-reversible, and those changes that are common in advanced age, that are not a result of the aging process, but of disease processes (Shay, 2000). Normal changes as a result of aging that occur to structures within the mouth are difficult to describe in the strictest sense because many other factors affect the teeth and the related supporting tissues, including a lifetime of mechanical, thermal (hot, cold, or frozen foods and beverages), and other environmental challenges to a patient's teeth (Shay, 2000). However, one can describe frequently occurring changes in the intact and functional teeth of the older individual. It is important to note that tooth loss, periodontal (gum) disease, and the loss of smell, hearing, or taste are not necessarily part of the normal aging process, but are symptoms of disease processes that must be addressed by the health care professional. Furthermore, these conditions can have a negative impact not only on appearance, but also on the patient's nutritional status by compromising his or her interest in and ability to properly chew a wide variety of foods (Tepper, 2001). The negative outcome has been known to be severe digestive problems or even choking (Schwartz, 2000).

The enamel of the tooth undergoes both chemical and morphological (shape) changes over time. Although enamel is the hardest human tissue, its composition becomes less hydrated and undergoes superficial increases in fluorine content with age, especially if the patient has been exposed regularly to fluoride through toothpaste and fluoridation of drinking water (Shay, 2000). Other changes to the external tooth structure occur such as changes in form from wear and attrition, and changes in tooth color, a gradual yellowing or darkening of teeth, due to both enamel wear and to changes in the quality and quantity of dentin, the insulating layer between the enamel and the pulp. Also, over the life of the tooth, a gradual increase in the amount of cementum, the material covering the root of the tooth, occurs. There are changes to the internal structure of a tooth as well, such as a decrease in the size of the root canal from the increase in dentin laid down inside the pulp (nerve) chamber as a result of age and in response to cavities, and a decrease in the ability of the pulp to repair itself. (Mjör, 1986).

There are also changes to the soft tissue, such as the cheeks, gums, lips, and tongue, including a thinning and smoothing of the lining of the mouth, a loss of elasticity, and an increase in susceptibility to mechanical injury (such as from tooth brushing, tobacco use, or biting), much as occurs to the appearance and resilience of the skin as a person ages (Mackenzie, Holm-Pedersen, & Karri, 1986). Additionally, there are changes to periodontal tissues (tissues of the gum that support the teeth), all of which may affect the functional and resilient properties of these tissues (Mackenzie, et al.).

Saliva is critical to preserving oral health. It does so by aiding in the preparation and movement of chewed food, lubricating the lining of the mouth, helping to preserve the oral microbial balance, cleansing the oral cavity, assisting with antibacterial and antimicrobial properties, assisting in keeping the calcium in the enamel, maintaining oral pH to help in the prevention of cavities, and aiding in taste perception (Baum, Caruso, Ship, & Wolff, 1991). Saliva protects the oral cavity, the upper airway, and the digestive tract. It also facilitates many sensorimotor phenomena, such as swallowing and tongue mobility (Baum, et al.).

With age, there is some atrophy of the tissues that secrete saliva in the salivary glands, as well as degenerative changes in both the major and the minor salivary glands. However, there does not appear to be a significant decrease in the volume of saliva produced, possibly due to a functional reserve capacity of the glands. Saliva secretion is essential for normal health and function, and, while there are age-related changes to the composition of the salivary glands, there is no apparent alteration in either output or composition of saliva in healthy older persons (Baum et al.).

There are three distinct phases of normal swallowing: oral, pharyngeal, and esophageal. Oral motor function is responsible for the oral phase, but change in any of the three phases of swallowing may disrupt nutritional intake and place the individual at higher risk for choking or aspiration. However, in healthy adults, the normal aging process has clinically insignificant changes in the sensory, muscular, and neurological functions associated with swallowing (Ship & Chavez, 2000).

As with other body tissues, the dental tissues of older persons are different from those of younger persons. This presents a difficulty with restorative materials in that these materials that were developed for and tested in the mouths of younger individuals, may not perform in the same manner in an older mouth (Shay, 2000). As the older population increases with time, there will most likely be a demand for materials to be developed specifically for the older patient's oral health and well-being.

## NON–AGE-RELATED CHANGES TO ORAL HEALTH

The changes common with advanced age include non-normative alterations to the patient's physical status, such as a decline in locomotor activities and cognition; changes in vision, hearing, and speech; tooth loss due to untreated disease, cavities, or poor oral hygiene; and issues of polypharmacy (the use of multiple prescribed and/or over-the-counter medications). These changes are not related to the aging process per se, but may be a result of disease progression, disease treatments, malnutrition, and untreated disease.

In addition to these health changes, there are changes that may occur in the patient's living arrangements as physical and/or mental disabilities progress, which may have a negative effect on the oral health of the patient. These changes might include entering a long-term care or assisted living facility, moving in with family members, as well as remaining within one's own home, living alone, living with an aging spouse or companion or with health care provided either formally or informally. All of these changes may affect not only the oral health of the patient and the delivery of oral health care to the patient, but also the patient's general health and well-being. An association has been found between the loss of teeth due to periodontal disease and such diseases as atherosclerosis (cholesterol deposits on the walls of arteries), heart failure, ischemic heart disease (angina), and joint diseases (Berg et al., 2000).

Financial considerations with respect to the ability to pay for care may be a significant factor in treatment planning for the older adult as only 14.5% of seniors have dental insurance and most must pay out of pocket for dental care (Pyle & Stoller, 2003). However, the ability or lack thereof by older patients to afford to pay for dental treatment should not be presumed and must be explored in a sensitive manner as treatment plan options are prepared (Berg et al., 2000). Furthermore, the lack of inclusion of oral health care services under the Medicare program has contributed to the problem of access to care for older adults as the dental profession has remained independent from this federal program (Pyle & Stoller, 2003).

There may be a blurring of the distinction between normal aging and degenerative changes in the oral cavity due to the severity and frequency of thermal, physical, and chemical changes as well as other environmental factors that occur in the mouth and may have cumulative effects over time (Shay, 2000). The two different processes, environment and aging, might be responsible for an "aging" outcome in the mouth as it may help to explain the variability of presentation between individuals of the same chronological age with different oral ages (Shay, 2000). One notable change in oral demographics that has occurred in the current generation of older people is that they have retained more of their natural teeth compared with previous generations of older people. This has led to a higher risk for development of serious systemic diseases that may be derived from untreated dental problems (Tepper, 2001), especially aspiration pneumonia (Ship & Chavez, 2000) and other lung infections (MacEntee, 2000) that are related to poor oral hygiene and periodontal disease (Ship & Chavez, 2000).

The older person with natural teeth remains at higher risk for dental disease, most notably cavities and gum disease, as well as for the soft tissue pathology that may also affect those without natural teeth. In addition, dental disease experience, tooth loss, medical conditions, and medications add to the complexity of planning and treatment of these patients. Furthermore, the elderly have a disproportional amount of oral disease, possibly related to access to care issues (Pyle & Stoller, 2003).

## FUNCTIONAL ABILITY EFFECTS ON ORAL CARE

A large proportion of older persons are afflicted with one or more chronic conditions, and in the older-old, many will exhibit multiple chronic conditions. These conditions, including arthritis, heart disease, hearing impairments, orthopedic impairments, vision impairments, and diabetes, may have a direct impact on the type of care to be provided to the patient. It is important to assess these factors in providing treatment that can have a significant impact on outcome. Clinical assessment of the type and severity of the patient's dental needs, the patient's ability to withstand the stresses of treatment, and the functional capability of the patient and his or her resources for the maintenance of oral health following treatment should all be considerations in the type and scope of treatment to be provided. Also, the concerns and perceived needs of the patient should be addressed to indicate the most appropriate levels of care and the best treatment options for the individual (Berg et al., 2000).

The older person's functional and mental capabilities to maintain restorations (fillings and crowns), prostheses (partial or full dentures), and periodontal health successfully are all critical elements in treatment planning. One should consider the person's perceived motivation for and ability to perform home oral health care such as flossing and brushing. Another consideration is whether there are resources such as family, friends, or others available to assist with or perform essential oral care if the individual has functional impairments that may compromise the ability to perform oral care alone (Berg et al., 2000). For persons with chronic disease(s), it is important to understand the role of the disease or diseases in their daily life. For example, a majority of persons over the age of 70 suffer from arthritis. If the arthritis is in the upper extremities, or is particularly deforming, such as rheumatoid arthritis, it may greatly hinder the ability to perform daily oral health care. In cases of debilitating arthritides and as visual acuity decreases, assistive devices such as electric toothbrushes, grip adaptors, flossing aids, and oral irrigation devices may increase the long-term success of dental treatment (Niessen & Gibson, 2000; Ship & Chavez, 2000). Deterioration in the person's functional abilities, both physical and cognitive, may increase the difficulty of receiving dental care, either in the dental office or in the long-term care facility (Niessen & Gibson, 2000). Chronic diseases that afflict older adults commonly and those treatments that mitigate the impact of such diseases on activities of daily living may affect the health and care of the oral cavity (Shay, 2000).

Altered chewing behaviors are frequently reported in older persons. This has been noted in both older people with intact teeth, and those who are partially or completely without teeth. This can often result in the inadequate preparation of food before swallowing (Ship & Chavez, 2000).

## XEROSTOMIA

The reduction or absence of saliva flow, known as xerostomia or dry mouth, has many serious consequences to the elderly (Baum et al., 1991). The most common cause of xerostomia is medication consumption. Other causes include autoimmune disease, which affects the physical structure of the salivary gland (Sjögren's Syndrome), radiation therapy, and chemotherapy. Sreebny and Schwartz (1997) reported that of the 200 most prescribed drugs in 1992, 63% potentially could cause dry mouth symptoms. While the actual mechanism for xerostomia from medication use is not well understood, some medications, such as anti-cholinergics, are known to reduce salivary flow, and others may dehydrate oral tissues, resulting in the feeling of dryness (Niessen & Gibson, 2000). Dry mouth is a very common potential side effect of a large proportion of prescription medications used in the older population. The scant or absent saliva may predispose the teeth to a buildup of plaque, increased cavities, and both new and recurrent decay, due to the lack of the natural buffering action of saliva, loss of tooth structure on the biting and grinding surfaces due to excessive wear, and mucosal disease (Shay, 2000), as well as an increase in halitosis (bad breath). The increase in dental cavities also depends upon whether there is pre-existing periodontal disease present. This may cause an increase in cavities on the now exposed tooth root due to recession of the gums, since the root is covered with cementum, which is softer and less mineralized than enamel. There will also be an increase in cavities of the crown of the tooth.

## ACCESS TO DENTAL CARE IN LONG-TERM CARE FACILITIES

As the number of older people living in long-term care facilities at some time in their lives increases, combined with declining incidence of tooth loss in this population, there will be an increased need to provide dental services within the long-term care facility (An, Douglass, & Monopoli,

2003). Institutionalized persons or those in assisted living environments may experience much higher levels of oral diseases as they generally may not be capable of performing self-administered oral care and are dependent on a caregiver for oral hygiene (Janket, Jones, Rich, Meurman, Garcia, & Miller, 2003). Residents with dementia or other psychiatric conditions present behavioral challenges that complicate oral health in that they may be too frightened, uncomprehending, or combative to permit oral hygiene procedures or dental treatments (Schwartz, 2000). It is worth noting that as health status declines such that a patient becomes homebound or enters a facility, the patient's oral health status declines as well. In this population, edentulism (loss of teeth) and cavity rates vary widely, but exceed the national average for a healthy population (Niessen & Gibson, 2000). There is also a perceived lack of need by the patient, the patient's family or caregiver, and the nursing staff for oral health care, and the assumption by patients and caregivers that dental problems such as periodontal disease and tooth loss are part of the normal aging process, with a resulting reluctance to seek oral care (An et al., 2003). Additionally, given the prevalence of sugar-laden diets in society generally, the dietary selection in long-term care facilities may contain a large amount of refined carbohydrates. This may contribute to the occurrence of cavities in this population, which may threaten to destroy the natural teeth of residents if there is a reliance only on oral health care and no control of diet constituents (MacEntee, 2000).

An and colleagues (2003) noted that there is a lack of integration of medical and dental care services in long-term care facilities that can affect the maintenance of oral health. The most satisfactory arrangement in the provision of oral care to long-term care residents involves the dental personnel as integral players on the health care team, and, in particular, as full participants in care conferences regularly convened to assess each resident (MacEntee, 2000). Furthermore, although physicians, nurses, aides, and other medical providers have regular contact with the residents, the providers' ability to recognize oral health problems is often limited (An et al., 2003).

An and colleagues (2003) listed the following four "Goals for Nursing Home Dental Care" as developed by the American Society for Geriatric Dentistry:

1.  Oral health care should be provided to prevent disease, maintain chewing and speaking ability, and preserve comfort, hygiene, and dignity.

2. Both the standard of oral health care and access to it should be equal to that in the community at large.
3. Residents or their representatives should have the right to choose (1) whether or not to receive oral health care, (2) who will provide their care, and (3) what specific oral health services will be provided.
4. All caregivers should advocate against the neglect of oral health problems suffered by vulnerable adults who cannot advocate for themselves.

All decisions for treatment should place the welfare of the patient first, taking into account the patient's tolerance for procedures and abilities to maintain oral care (Goldstein & Mulligan, 1991). By offering an accessible monitoring, diagnostic, and treatment service directly to elders in long-term care, and by educating the nursing staff to offer daily oral health care as an integral part of personal hygiene for all patients, there will most likely be a reduction in the risk of morbidity and mortality in long-term care facilities. This may also contribute to successful aging of patients by improving their quality of life (MacEntee, 2000).

## NON-INSTITUTIONAL CARE OF DISABLED ELDERS

Approximately 10% of the senior population is disabled, but homebound, and not institutionalized. Delivering oral health care to these patients is of concern.

Some of the oral health care access problems for patients in long-term care apply to the homebound senior as well. As the homebound senior becomes more reliant on spouse, family members, or friends for assistance and not on trained health care providers, their levels of oral disease may be at the same or even higher level as those patients in long-term care facilities. Domiciliary dental care may benefit the population of elderly with mobility problems and those with cognitive disorders, such as dementia or Alzheimer's disease, who, while physically able to visit the dental office, become disoriented and confused in unfamiliar environments (Fiske, 2000). Although there is substantial demand for oral health care by the homebound elderly, it is less than the actual need. Elderly patients with diminished mental capacity may not even be aware that they have oral disease (Goldstein & Mulligan, 1991).

Treatment plans for elderly patients may be complicated by barriers to care such as mobility or cognitive problems, disease, uncertainty about benefits and risks for the patient, and an inadequate knowledge about patient preferences with respect to treatment (Pyle & Stoller, 2003). The goal for optimal care should not be automatically aimed toward the highest technically possible level but toward the highest appropriate level of care for a specific patient's needs (Berg et al., 2000). Paying for dental care is a growing concern, particularly for a large segment of the U.S. older population (Berg et al., 2000).

## CONCLUSIONS

Oral health care is an important issue in our society, and barriers to its delivery to older patients must be eliminated. Older adults should expect to maintain or improve their oral health by improving the attractiveness of their smile, minimizing oral discomfort, and continuing or improving their ability to chew a wide range of foods properly (Berg et al., 2000). Based on the numbers and proportion of the older population compared with the entire population, their increased retention of teeth, the impact of chronic medical conditions and their treatment on oral health, and the associations between dental and systemic diseases, the dental health care provider of tomorrow must be prepared to face the unique challenges of an aging population in the practice of general dentistry (Pyle & Stoller, 2003). Given that there are numerous unmet dental needs in the older population, both in the institutionalized and the non-institutionalized, attention must be focused on remedying the current situation and preparing for the projected increase in this population as the baby boomers begin to enter their golden years. Because people over the age of 65 are the fastest growing segment of the population and will continue to grow as the baby boomers start to enter this age group, dental concerns will need to be addressed and incorporated into general health care. Older people will demand better oral health care in terms of prevention and treatment options. Older people are retaining more of their natural teeth and are interested in maintaining their appearance and functional ability, in addition to preserving their health. This has already led to an awareness on the part of the dental profession to provide specialized care for this population and specialized dental education for students and dental practitioners alike.

## REFERENCES

An, G., Douglass, C. W., & Monopoli, M. (2003). Considerations for dental treatment in long-term care facilities. *Journal of the Massachusetts Dental Society, 52*(1), 28–32.

Baum, B. J., Caruso, A. J., Ship, J. A., & Wolff, A. (1991). Oral physiology. In A. S. Pappas, L. C. Niessen, & H. H. Chauncey (Eds.), *Geriatric dentistry: Aging and oral health* (pp. 71–82). St. Louis: Mosby-Year Book.

Berg, R., Garcia, L. T., & Berkey, D. B. (2000). Spectrum of care treatment planning: Application of the model in older adults. *General Dentistry, Sept.–Oct.,* 534–543.

Fiske, J. (2000). The delivery of oral care services to elderly people living in noninstitutionalized settings. *Journal of Public Health Dentistry, 60*(4), 321–325.

Goldstein, C. M., & Mulligan, R. (1991). Delivering treatment to the confined elderly. In A. S. Pappas, L. C. Niessen, & H. H. Chauncey (Eds.), *Geriatric dentistry: Aging and oral health* (pp. 285–308). St. Louis: Mosby-Year Book.

Janket, S.-J., Jones, J. A., Rich, S., Meurman, J., Garcia, R., & Miller, D. (2003). Xerostomic medications and oral health: The veterans dental study (Part I). *Gerodontology, 20*(1), 41–49.

MacEntee, M. I. (2000). Oral care for successful aging in long-term care. *Journal of Public Health Dentistry, 60*(4), 326–329.

Mackenzie, I. C., Holm-Pedersen, P., & Karring, T. (1986). Age changes in the oral mucous membranes and periodontium. In P. Holm-Pederson & H. Löe (Eds.), *Geriatric dentistry* (pp. 102–113). Copenhagen: Munksgaard.

Mjör, I. A. (1986). Age changes in the teeth. In P. Holm-Pederson & H. Löe (Eds.), *Geriatric dentistry* (pp. 94–101). Copenhagen: Munksgaard.

Niessen, L. C., & Gibson, G. (2000). Aging and oral health for the 21st century. *General Dentistry, Sept.–Oct.,* 544–549.

Pyle, M. A., & Stoller, E. P. (2003). Oral health disparities among the elderly: Interdisciplinary challenges for the future. *Journal of Dental Education, 67*(12), 1327–1336.

Schwartz, M. (2000). The oral health of the long-term care patient. *Annals of Long-Term Care: Clinical Care and Aging, 8*(12), 41–46.

Shay, K. (2000). Restorative considerations in the dental treatment of the older patient. *General Dentistry, Sept.–Oct.,* 550–554.

Ship, J. A., & Chavez, E. M. (2000). Management of systemic diseases and chronic impairments in older adults: Oral health considerations. *General Dentistry, Sept.–Oct.,* 555–565.

Sreebny, L. M., & Schwartz, S. S. (1997). A reference guide to drugs and dry mouth—2nd edition. *Gerodontology, 14*(1), 33–47.

Surgeon General's Report. (2000, May). *Oral Health in America: A Report of the Surgeon General.* Rockville, MD: U.S. Department of Health and Human Services, National Institute of Dental and Craniofacial Research, National Institutes of Health.

Tepper, L. (2001). Paying attention to oral health. *City Health Information: The New York City Department of Health Summary of Reportable Diseases and Conditions, 1999, 20*(1), 7.

# 9

# Major Mental Disorders of Old Age

## Gary J. Kennedy

The major mental disorders account for the majority of older persons' disability and their associated family burden. Our understanding of the character, causes, and treatment of psychopathology in later life has advanced dramatically. This would not have been possible without the public's demand for better clinical training and more scientific research. Nonetheless the promise of better mental health in old age through clinical intervention remains largely unfulfilled. What follows are brief descriptions of the mental illnesses that most commonly afflict seniors. The goal is to increase awareness of the need to improve both the accessibility and acceptance of mental health care in late life.

### DEPRESSION AND ANXIETY

Symptoms of depression and anxiety are frequently seen together in late life. As a result, the disorders are more difficult to distinguish, diagnose, and treat than they are in younger persons. Although psychotherapeutic techniques for treating anxiety and depressive disorders differ, the choice of medications (antidepressants for either condition) and the approach to the course of illness are quite similar. Given the frequency with which depression and anxiety disorders go untreated when we consider the safety and efficacy of present interventions, practitioners are urged to lower the threshold for offering treatment.

A major change in the clinical approach to old age depression occurred in the 1990s (Karasu, Docherty, & Gelenberg, 1993), resulting in an expanse of therapeutic indications, treatments, outcomes, and endpoints that is best captured by the geriatric syndrome concept.

Geriatric syndromes such as cognitive impairment, gait disorder, and incontinence are signs or symptoms caused by a range of diagnoses such that a "sort out" rather than "rule out" approach is necessary to reduce the associated disability. The syndromal approach also resolves much of the conflict between epidemiological (Myers et al., 1984) and clinical studies of depression (Kermis, 1986) in old age. Epidemiologic studies find depressive symptoms pervasive but depressive disorders infrequent in older community residents. In medical clinic populations both symptoms and disorders are frequent. The symptoms may arise from bereavement, the despondency associated with recent onset disability, a perception of failing health, loss of hope as a result of confinement from agoraphobia, or a major depressive episode. As will be argued below, when symptoms do not conform to diagnostic criteria for a major mental disorder, they may yet be associated with genuine disability, which is in turn a legitimate focus of clinical attention.

## THE COEXISTENCE OF MENTAL AND PHYSICAL ILLNESS

As many as 30% of elderly primary-care patients demonstrate significant depressive symptomatology. Close to half that number meet criteria for a depressive disorder. Hypnotics and antianxiety agents are more often prescribed for older adults with depressive symptoms than are antidepressants. Not surprisingly, depressive symptoms tend to persist in the routine care context (Kennedy, Kelman, & Thomas, 1991). Depressive symptoms among older adults lead to utilization of outpatient services and nursing facilities (Kelman & Thomas, 1990) beyond that expected for the level of disability associated with their medical conditions. Depression amplifies physical disability, and even minor depression may be more disabling than many chronic physical conditions. As many as one quarter of those with minor depression experience a major depressive disorder within twenty-four months. More important, the disability of depression may be avoidable.

Major depression occurs in more than half of patients within six months following stroke (Parikh, Lipsey, & Robinson, 1987). Generalized anxiety disorder is also common in the post-stroke period with close to one quarter of patients meeting diagnostic criteria. Of those, three quarters will also meet criteria of major or minor depression (Schultz, Castillo, Kosier, & Robinson, 1997). Both anxiety and depression substantially interfere with rehabilitation. Twenty percent of Parkinson patients develop a major depressive episode, and twenty percent experience dysthymia (2 symptoms of depression occurring for 2 years), frequently combined with anxiety. Depressive symptoms are also common in dementia patients (Rovner, Broadhead, Spencer, Carson, & Folstein, 1989) and their caregiving family members in the community (Gallagher, Rose, Rivera, Losett, & Thompson, 1989). Dementia is the most prevalent mental illness in nursing homes, but depression, and dementia complicated by depression, are also frequently encountered (Rovner, German, Broadhead, et al., 1990).

Although older adults are more likely to develop a major depressive episode following bereavement than are younger adults, physical illness and disability explain substantially more of the variance in the prevalence and course of depressive symptoms than sociodemographic, life event, and interpersonal factors do (Kennedy, Kelman, Thomas, Wisniewski, Metz, & Bijur, 1989). Katz (1996) summarizes two general theories regarding the biological origins of depression in late life. First, subclinical cerebrovascular disease may induce depressive symptoms through neurohumoral or structural brain changes. Indeed the profile of depressive symptoms in depression associated with vascular disease is characterized by motor retardation, lack of insight, and impaired executive (planning) function, suggesting frontal brain system dysfunction (Lebowitz et al., 1997). Second, systemic illness may induce depression through immunologic-mediated changes in behavior that allow the sick individual time to recover physiologic equilibrium by reducing activities related to sex and aggression.

## ANXIETY DISORDERS

The fourth edition of the *Diagnostic and Statistical Manual of Mental Disorders* (American Psychiatric Association, 1994) lists several Anxiety Disorders. They include Panic Disorder with and without Agoraphobia, Agoraphobia without history of panic, Social Phobia (Social Anxiety Disorder), Specific (Simple) Phobia, Obsessive-Compulsive Disorder, Generalized Anxiety Disorder, Anxiety Disorder Due to a General Medical Condition, Posttraumatic Stress Disorder (Chronic, Acute or Delayed Onset), and Acute Stress Disorder. Duration of symptoms and their temporal relation to the traumatic event distinguishes Posttraumatic from Acute Stress Disorder. Posttraumatic Disorder may arise at some distance from the event but lasts at least one month. Acute Stress Disorder arises within one month of the event and lasts from 2 days to one month. In either disorder the patient experiences intrusive recollections or images of the traumatic event, emotional numbing, recurrent nightmares, avoidance of stimuli associated with the traumatic event, hypervigilance, sleep disturbance, and irritability. These individuals relive the trauma and are substantially disabled as a result.

Among physically healthy older community residents without cognitive disorders, agoraphobia may be more common than depression, affecting 6% of women and 3.6% of men. Panic disorder and obsessive-compulsive disorder affect less than one percent each. Considering all anxiety disorders combined, women experience 6.8% prevalence, and men 3.6%. Minor depression and the mixed syndrome of depression with anxiety affect more than 1% of older community residents (Blazer et al., 1989). There is considerable comorbidity of depression with generalized anxiety disorder and phobias in older persons. Subsyndromal anxiety and anxiety occurring together with psychiatric and medical disorders are also significant (Smith, Sherrill, & Colenda, 1995). Anxiety may be evidence of poor recovery from a previous episode of depression (Blazer, Hughes, & Fowler, 1989).

The symptom profile of anxiety disorders in late life is similar to that seen at younger ages with the exception of obsessive-compulsive disorder in which "fear of having sinned" is more frequent in seniors (Kohn, Westlake, Rasmussen, Marsland, & Norman, 1997). Anxious persons are apprehensive, tense, and have a sense of dread. They may be irritable, startle easily, feel restless or on edge, and find it difficult to fall asleep. As with depression, they have physical symptoms. There are difficulties with gastrointestinal function including trouble swallowing, indigestion, excessive flatulence, and either too frequent or too few bowel movements. They may worry excessively about their health, their memory, their money, the safety of the neighborhood, falling, or being mugged while out of the house. Hyperthyroidism and congestive heart failure are chronic diseases that cause anxiety, as do steroids, thyroid hormone, caffeine, and ephedra.

Most older patients with panic disorder have experienced the onset early in life and have received little or no treatment (Sheikh, King, & Taylor, 1991). Not surprisingly, panic disorder tends to become chronic. Simple phobias, generalized anxiety disorder, and obsessive-compulsive disorder are commonly associated with panic disorder (American Psychiatric Association, 1994). Untreated panic attacks may lead to agoraphobia, depression, alcohol abuse (Kushner, Sher, & Beitman, 1990), and suicide. Of those who are treated, the mainstay anxiolytic has been a benzodiazepine. Benzodiazepines are sedative, impair cognition, put the person at risk for a fall, and are difficult to withdraw. Of note, 11% of men and 25% of women aged 60–74 use anxiolytics; individuals aged 65 and older consume 21% of all benzodiazepine prescriptions. Older adults taking long-acting benzodiazepines experience excess numbers of motor vehicle accidents (Hemmelgarn, Suissa, Huang, Boivin, &

Pinard, 1997). In summary, the bulk of evidence indicates that when generalized anxiety and depression are concurrent, the primary diagnosis in late life is a depressive disorder whether encountered in the community, clinic (Blazer, Hughes, & Fowler, 1989) or in the nursing home.

## THE DEMENTIAS

There are 4 million Americans afflicted with dementia at a cost near $100 billion a year. The indirect or hidden expense to the family members providing care is estimated to be an additional $100 billion. With the number of persons with dementia projected to double over the next 40 years (Ernst & Hay, 1994), even modest benefits to the individual will have a substantial cost offset if achieved in the population at large. Advances in the treatment of cognitive impairment and the genetic detection of individuals at risk before onset of the disease promise a genuine breakthrough.

### Dementia Defined

All dementias share three elements. First is progressive decline, which differentiates dementia from developmental disorders that emerge in childhood but remain stable throughout adult life. Second is compound rather than circumscribed impairment of cognition. Persons with dementia have learning and memory problems plus at least one of the following: impairments in the ability to communicate, to reason and plan, to manipulate objects in space, to be oriented, alert, and to modulate emotion. This distinguishes dementia from the pure disorders of memory and the nonprogressive disorders of communication seen in the aphasias and stroke. Third, dementia in the early and middle stages does not impair consciousness, which separates it from delirium. Dementia is a general complex of symptoms, which may also be part of an etiologically specific disorder as in neurosyphilis. In summary, it is a syndrome of progressive and global decline in cognitive capacities, severe enough to substantially interfere with the individual's well-being and social function.

### The Epidemiology of Dementia

Because dementia is an age-related disorder, as the proportion of older adults increases both the incidence and prevalence of dementia will increase. Alzheimer's disease alone affects 8 to 15 percent of persons 65 or older. But among individuals 85 and older, more than 15% are severely demented, with the prevalence approaching 50% among those with a demented first-degree relative (Mohs, Breitner, Silverman, & Davis, 1987). The prevalence of dementia increases exponentially, doubling every 5 years at least to age 85. The wide variation in prevalence by gender, nationality, and ethnicity is poorly understood. The higher prevalence among women reflects their survival advantage over men rather than a higher incidence of the illness. And despite improved survival rates associated with cardiovascular disease, an increase in vascular-related dementia may be expected even if present cases are over diagnosed (Small et al., 1997). Educationally disadvantaged minorities may also be disproportionately affected by the increasing prevalence of dementia (Lilienfeld & Perl, 1994).

## Diagnostic Criteria

Although a histological examination of brain tissues sets the criteria for "definite" in Alzheimer's disease, the diagnosis of "probable" Alzheimer's dementia can be accurately made in 90% of cases by history from the patient and family and clinical examination (Small et al., 1997). "Possible" cases may have atypical features but no identifiable alternative diagnosis.

The nomenclature of dementia is confusing because of its historical origins and successful efforts to distinguish and separate types of the illness from the syndrome. The diagnosis is challenging particularly in the early stage because there are no definitive biological markers, the onset is often insidious, and other reversible causes of cognitive impairment either resemble or accompany dementia. Delirium is perhaps the most common cognitive disorder. The hallmarks are waxing and waning symptoms, impaired attention, visual hallucinations, and demonstrable physiologic disturbance. Symptoms should remit once the disturbance is reversed but recovery may be delayed in older persons, threatening a premature diagnosis of dementia. However persons with dementia are more susceptible to delirium. Delirium can also be chronic and difficult to distinguish from dementia.

Cognitive impairment due to depressive disorders is distinguished by the patient's prominent complaints of difficulty with memory and concentration. Apathy, irritability, and reluctance to complete cognitive testing are apparent but without aphasia (a disorder of language communication). The term "pseudodementia" was introduced in 1952 by

Madden and others who described cases in which the diagnosis of dementia was changed after a remission of cognitive deficits. Pseudo-dementia originally implied a misdiagnosis. However, present use of pseudodementia to describe the reversible cognitive impairment seen in late life depression leads to confusion and should be abandoned.

Age associated memory impairment (AAMI), or benign senescent forgetfulness is characterized by subjective memory complaints in persons age 50 or older whose performance falls by one standard deviation below the mean on formal memory tests normed for younger adults. Although lower memory scores are predictive of dementia, only 1–3% of these individuals will progress to global cognitive impairment (Richards, Touchon, Ledesert, & Richie, 1999). In contrast, 5–15% of persons with Mild Cognitive Impairment (MCI) will develop dementia in the coming year. MCI is characterized by memory performance between one and one-half standard deviation below the mean score of tests of memory. As with AAMI, persons with MCI have memory complaints but do not meet diagnostic criteria for dementia. They exhibit slowed information retrieval but orientation, communication, and functional independence are all intact. They also benefit from self-taught memory aides (Peterson, Smith, & Waring, 1999). Research trials are underway to determine if cholinesterase inhibitors (Aricept, Exelon, Reminyl), vitamin E, and anti-inflammatory agents prevent the progression of AAMI and MCI. A positive outcome with MCI would suggest it may simply be early dementia for which present diagnostic criteria are inadequate. The public health implications of early screening and intervention would be enormous.

Alzheimer's disease is the most frequently encountered dementia. The onset is insidious; the decline is smooth but more rapid in the middle stage in which behavioral disturbances start to emerge. Individuals with early Alzheimer's disease often minimize their deficits, unlike persons with MCI or depression.

Vascular dementias, characterized by brain cell degeneration, such as Multi-infarct and Binswanger's disease, are due to angiopathic disorders. Most commonly these are ischemic heart disease and arrhythmias (heart rhythm disorders), high blood pressure, and diabetes. Weakness in one side, gait disorder, and other signs of past stroke also suggest vascular dementia. However the pathology of vascular dementia is frequently of a mixed type (cortical and subcortical), with diverse presentations in which the loss of brain volume, ventricular dilatation, bradykinesia (slowed movement), and the cognitive deficits are difficult to distinguish from Alzheimer's disease.

Although perceptual distortions are common in dementia, when visual or auditory hallucinations are prominent, signs of Parkinson's

disease are evident, the onset was abrupt, and the course characterized
by lucid moments alternating with confusion, Lewy body disease may
be diagnosed (McKeith, Galasko, & Kosaka, 1996). Paranoid delusions,
falls, and depression are also characteristic of diffuse Lewy body
dementia.

The rare dementias would be easy to overlook were it not for their
distinctive features. Marked deficits in visual perception and praxis (the
capacity to manipulate objects in space) may suggest cortico-nuclear
degeneration. Early deterioration in personality, loss of social inhibi-
tions, and frontal lobe atrophy may indicate Pick's dementia (Heston,
White, & Mastri, 1987). Physical signs such as the tremor and bradykinesia of Parkinson's disease, the movement disorders of Huntington's
disease, the muscle twitching of Creutzfeldt-Jakob disease, or the
pseudo-bulbar palsy (difficulty swallowing) of vascular dementia may
present before intellectual deterioration is observed. Changes in affect
preceding signs of dementia, typically depression but also hypomania
and irritability, suggest a non-Alzheimer's diagnosis (Mahendra, 1985).
Huntington's disease is typical of the subcortical dementias in that
various cortical functions including communication, praxis, and visual
perception are generally spared. However memory impairment, apathy,
and psychomotor retardation are marked and progressive. Emotional
disturbances and personality change are regular features of Huntington's disease and frequently the first signs of the illness. Normal pressure
hydrocephalus is characterized by incontinence, abnormal (stuck to
the floor, or "magnetic") gait, and ventricular atrophy out of proportion
to cortical loss. The cognitive impairment of stroke or acute traumatic
brain injury may predispose the person to dementia but may also improve over the six months following the accident. Like the dementia
associated with the toxicity and nutritional deprivation of massive alcohol abuse, chronic injury in boxing and other contact sports and accidents is potentially preventable.

Dementia may also be secondary to infectious systemic disease such
as syphilis or acquired immune deficiency syndrome. Transmissible
disorders of the prion type (Creuztfeld-Jakob disease) may also cause
dementia through exposure to infected foods ("Mad Cow Disease") or
transplanted tissues or tissue extracts. Thus dementia may be classified
as infectious or transmissible. However, Katzman's (1986) more productive clinical nomenclature describes the dementias as reversible, irrevers-
ible, or partially reversible. Although few dementias are reversible, most
have elements that will partially remit.

Staging of dementia is also important in that the cognitive enhancer
medications (see below) are FDA approved only for mild to moderate

Alzheimer's disease. Nonetheless many practitioners, patients or their families are comfortable with "off label" (non-traditional) use in cases of mild cognitive impairment, vascular, and Lewy body dementias and late stage Alzheimer's disease. Patients with Mini Mental Status Examination (MMSE) scores above 20 are classified with mild Alzheimer's dementia. Their symptoms are characterized by memory loss and disorientation, repetitiousness, loss of interests, and change in personality. Although depression may appear early, delusions, agitation, sleep disturbance, and wandering are more characteristic of moderate dementia. Persons with moderately advanced dementia have MMSE scores ranging between 10 and 19. They require supervision to complete tasks of daily living such as dressing and to be safe from dangerous wandering. Patients with MMSE scores of 9 and under are diagnosed with severe dementia, evidenced by marked speech disorders, loss of capacity to recognize family, incontinence, and dependency in all aspects of daily living. Stated simply, mildly impaired persons are forgetful and sometimes disoriented but can care for most of their personal needs. Moderately impaired persons require supervision for care and safety. Severely impaired persons are totally dependent and are losing the capacity to recognize family.

## PSYCHOSIS AND MANIA IN LATE LIFE

Treatment options for psychotic disorders and mania have improved considerably in the last decade, offering a more optimistic prognosis. The observation that deterioration following psychosis is not inevitable has brought about new enthusiasm for both treatment and research. But the similarities between late onset schizophrenia, delusional disorder, mania, and the psychoses of depression, dementia, and stroke can make the diagnosis difficult among older adults. Compounding the diagnostic problem is the overlap between the psychotic disorders and psychotic episodes seen in individuals with personality disorders who are transiently overwhelmed by stressful events.

### The Schizophrenias

Although the burden of dementia is substantial, the premature mortality and total years lost in personal productivity and autonomy make schizophrenia the most devastating mental illness of adult life. The prevalence is 1% in both the developed and developing nations. Close to 2 million people are treated for the illness every year with upwards of 100,000 in hospitals every day. Sixty percent of affected individuals will receive disability benefits within the first year of onset. Ten percent will commit suicide within that first year. The majority of those who survive will neither marry nor have children (Andreasen, 1999). For patients young or old, the critical elements of successful treatment are a comprehensive, individualized approach including medication, family support and education, and aggressive case management outreach, known as assertive community management for persons at high risk for hospitalization. Although 90% of persons with schizophrenia receive antipsychotic medication, only 50% receive the recommended array of psychosocial and rehabilitative services. Failure to add an antidepressant medication for depressive episodes and failure to provide for psychosocial treatments (family intervention, therapeutic day programs) are the most frequent inadequacies. States vary in the availability of therapeutic programs. Yet the failure to treat depression, which is no less common in persons with schizophrenia than anyone else, should be more easily remedied. Until recently, schizophrenia was seen as an illness starting in the young adult years. Social and intellectual deterioration was inevitable. By late life the prevalence of schizophrenia in the community was thought to be less than one percent as a result of premature mortality and premature dementia, resulting in nursing home admission. More recent data suggest that schizophrenic psychoses are more prevalent in late life but do not inevitably lead to dementia (Jeste, Symonds, & Harris, 1997). A number of clinical scientists now argue that schizophrenia can have a distinct late onset form, occurring between ages 45 and 60. Although most cases of schizophrenia in males occur in the second and third decades of life, the illness demonstrates a bimodal age of onset among women, with a significant second peak occurring in the menopausal years (Häfner, 1997; Jeste et al., 1997). The loss of initiative and blunted emotionality persist, whereas delusions and hallucinations diminish with age. The result is a more varied course, including return of capacity for independent living in a significant minority of persons in middle age (Cohen, 1995). Nonetheless, older persons with schizophrenia experience a quality of life similar to that of dementia patients and generate increased health care costs compared to their younger peers (Cuffel, Jeste, Patterson, Halpain, & Pratt, 1997).

Late onset schizophrenia resembles early onset disease in several ways. The positive symptoms are more prominent in women; impairments in visual and auditory processing are common, as is a family history of psychosis and a personal history of adjustment problems in childhood. Sensory impairments, particularly hearing difficulties, which were thought to contribute to the onset of paranoia, may be the result of difficulty acquiring and accommodating to glasses and hearing aids caused by the illness. The overall pattern of cognitive impairment is similar in early and late onset disease, as are findings of non-specific white matter and ventricular abnormalities on brain MRI. The course is persistent, and mortality is increased. Late onset disease, is more frequent in women, shows less severe negative symptoms, and is mostly delusional and paranoid in character. Impairments in learning, abstraction, and cognitive flexibility are not as severe. Most important, favorable responses are obtained at lower doses of antipsychotics, although full remission of symptoms is rare.

## Delusional Disorder

In Delusional (Paranoid) Disorder, false beliefs and inferences seriously impair social judgment and cannot be interpreted as originating from religious or cultural group norms. Pathological suspiciousness, jealousy, exaggerated self-regard, and erotic obsession are the most frequent manifestations. Most aspects of personality and cognitive performance remain intact. However failure to pay bills, neglect of physical illness or disability, and accusations against others for which there is little or no basis in fact bring these people to the attention of social service agencies. Antipsychotic medication will in most instances substantially restore the person's capacity to manage, but only one in four will abandon the delusions and gain clear insight into their difficulties.

## Mania

Late onset mania is often misdiagnosed and as a result is likely to be more common than previously reported. The presentation is more complex and less typical of classical bipolar (manic depressive) illness. Diagnostic certainty is often clouded by the presence of cognitive impairment suggesting dementia. Late onset mania is more often secondary or closely associated in etiology to other medical disorders, most commonly stroke, dementia, or hyperthyroidism, but also medications including antidepressants, steroids, estrogens, and other agents with known central nervous system properties (Young, Moline, & Kleyman, 1997). The prognosis is generally less favorable than for earlier onset mania. A careful history from the family may uncover repeated hypomanic episodes that did not seriously impair the individual but in retrospect are clear indicators of early onset disease. The difficulties of recognizing the diagnosis, treatment of contributing conditions, age-related vulnerability to medication side effects, and the frequency with which structural brain changes, which frequently include subcortical hyperintensities seen on MRI, are associated all make treatment more difficult (McDonald, Krishnan, Doraiswamy, & Blazer, 1996).

Late onset mania is more frequently seen among men than women. The manic episode often presents with confusion, disorientation, distractibility, and irritability rather than elevated, positive mood. Conversely, the clinical interview may be characterized by irrelevant content delivered with an argumentative, intense, yet fluent quality. Patently unrealistic plans concerning finances or travel, exaggerated self-regard, and contentious claims to certainty in the face of evidence to the contrary are also seen. The statements may be plausible rather than bizarre but are too improbable to be real. The unsuspecting examiner is often puzzled by the difficulty of the interchange until the diagnosis of mania is considered.

## SUICIDE

Sociologists and journalists assert that the increase in late life suicides reflects elder fears of dependency, nursing home, and unwanted invasive care (Angell, 1990). In contrast, clinical scientists argue that depression and brain chemistry disturbances are the driving force behind late life suicide (Mann & Stoff, 1997). Chronic illness, alcoholism, and the availability of firearms (Marzuk, Leon, Tardiff, Morgan, Marina, & Mann, 1992) have also been cited, as well as a greater social acceptance of suicide among the elderly (Grabbe, Demi, Camann, & Potter, 1997). However this apparent antagonism between biomedical and sociological causes indicates much about desirable interventions.

### Suicide Rates in Later Life

The highest rates of suicide are found in the elderly, ranging from less than 3 in 100,000 among African-American women, to more than 60 in 100,000 among white males entering their ninth decade (Public Health Service, 2001). At present rates, which have remained stable for more than 10 years, the number of deaths due to suicide among older persons will double over the next 40 years. Both social (Durkheim, 1951) and psychopathological (Conwell, Melanie, & Caine, 1990) factors contribute to suicidal vulnerability. Precisely how biomedical and sociodemographic factors interact to increase the risk of late life suicide is unclear.

### Trends in the Prevalence of Late Life Suicide

By 1987 the rate of 21.6 suicides per 100,000 older adults exceeded that at the 1965 inception of Medicare. This was a reverse in the downward trend in elderly suicide that began in 1933 (Kennedy, Metz, & Lowinger, 1996). The rate of late life suicides increased despite advances in the economic and health status of older adults. Suicide is the tenth leading cause of death among older adults and the third most common cause of death from injury following falls and automobile accidents (Grabbe et al., 1997). Close to 6,000 seniors kill themselves each year, accounting for one third of all suicides. Present rates, based on death certificates and family reports, are an underestimate of actual suicide rate (Miller, 1978). Survivors' guilt over missing the warning signs biases reports toward calling them accidents rather than suicides. For every completed late life suicide there are at least four attempts. The number of physically ill isolated older adults who commit suicide through self-neglect is unknown. Public opinion polls suggest that as many as 600,000 adults aged 60 or older have considered suicide over a 6-month period (Gallup, 1992). If the percentage of older suicides increases no further, the number of late life suicides will double over the next 40 years (Whanger, 1989).

### Gender, Race, and Social Factors

Male gender is a risk factor regardless of age. Above age 65, 80% of suicides are male (United States Public Health Service, 1999). The preponderance of white males among elderly suicides has been the case since the turn of the century, but suicide rates in African-American men have also increased since 1968. Explanations for the high rates of elderly suicide, particularly in older white males, include divorce and loss of status related to retirement. The rate for divorced men is 3.2 times that for married men and 18.9 that for married women (Meehan, Saltzberg, & Sattir, 1991).

### Physical Illness

Among individuals 60 years of age and older, as many as 70 percent may have had a physical illness directly contributing to the completion of suicide. Diseases of the heart, lung, and central nervous system are frequently cited (Horton-Deustch, Clark, & Farran, 1992). Clark (1992) found 20% of older persons committing suicide had visited their physician within one day of death. Their physicians recalled patient presentations of vague physical complaints and denial of mental symptoms when specifically questioned. In contrast, their families reported depression and problems with alcohol and prescription medications. Some late life suicides result from a perception of terminal illness that cannot be verified by medical examination. However it is unclear that these distorted perceptions are delusions or simply an expression of hopelessness, which has often been linked to suicidality (Beck, Steer, Kovacs, & Garrison, 1985).

## Mental Disorders and Suicide

Studies of psychiatric patients indicate that a depressive episode is present in from two thirds to 90% of older adults who commit suicide (Conwell et al., 1990). Severity of depressive symptoms, rather than the presence of psychosis, correlates with completed suicide. However, information from community samples suggests that depressive disorders may play a less prominent role in late life suicide. Weissman and others reported the frequency of suicidal thoughts and a history of suicide attempts among participants in the Epidemiologic Catchment Area studies (Weissman, Klerman, Markowitz, & Ouellette, 1989). Surprisingly, no relationship between depressive disorder and suicide attempts or suicidal thoughts was observed. Panic attacks and panic disorders, but not advanced age, were related to suicidal ideas and attempts. Although not all older adults who express suicidal ideas attempt suicide, it is thought that most elderly suicides have verbalized the thought. Based on mortality statistics and survey data, at least 5% of older persons have thought of suicide in the last year but only 1% of that number will have died of suicide. Thus some measure of suicidal thinking such as that found in instruments like the Zung Self-Rating Depression Scale (1985) or the Hamilton Depression Rating Scale (1960) is worth incorporating when the risk profile or clinical suspicions run high.

## CONCLUSION

Scientific advances in etiology, diagnosis, and treatment continue to accelerate, as does the public's acceptance of treatment and expectations for benefits. However, the mental health delivery system continues to be less than adequate and far from ideal. Major changes in mental health financing policies and in clinical practice will be necessary if the scientific promise of mental health in old age is to be realized.

## REFERENCES

American Psychiatric Association. (1994). *Diagnostic and statistical manual of mental disorders* (4th ed.). Washington, DC: Author.

Andreasen, N. (1999). Understanding the causes of schizophrenia. *New England Journal of Medicine, 430,* 645–647.

Angell, M. (1990). Prisoners of technology: The case of Nancy Cruzan. *New England Journal of Medicine, 322,* 1226–1228.

Beck, A. T., Steer, R. A., Kovacs, M., & Garrison, B. (1985). Hopelessness and eventual suicide: A 10-year prospective study of patients hospitalized with suicidal ideation. *American Journal of Psychiatry, 142,* 559–563.

Blazer, D. G., Hughes, D. C., & Fowler, N. (1989). Anxiety as an outcome of depression in the elderly and middle-aged. *International Journal of Geriatric Psychiatry, 4,* 273–277.

Blazer, D., Woodbury, M., Hughes, D. C., George, L. K., Manton, K. G., Bachar, J. R., Fowler, N., & Cohen, H. J. (1989). A statistical analysis of the classification of depression in a mixed community and clinical sample. *Journal of Affective Disorders, 16,* 11–20.

Clark, D. C. (1992, December 10). Remarks presented at the "Too Young to Die" Conference on the National Suicide Survey conducted by Empire Blue Cross and Blue Shield and the Gallup Organization, Inc., New York.

Cohen, C. I. (1995). Studies of the course and outcome of schizophrenia in later life. *Psychiatric Services, 46,* 877–889.

Conwell, Y., Melanie, R., & Caine, E. D. (1990). Completed suicide at age 50 and over. *Journal of the American Geriatric Society, 38,* 640–644.

Cuffel, B. J., Jeste, D. V., Patterson, T. L., Halpain, M., & Pratt, C. (1997). Treatment costs and use of community mental health services for schizophrenia by age-cohorts. *American Journal of Psychiatry, 153,* 870–876.

Durkheim, E. (1951). *Suicide.* New York: Free Press.

Ernst, R. L., & Hay, J. W. (1994). The U.S. economic and social costs of Alzheimer's disease revisited. *American Journal of Public Health, 84,* 1261–1264.

Gallagher, D., Rose, J., Rivera, P., Losett, S., & Thompson, L. W. (1989). Prevalence of depression in family caregivers. *Gerontologist, 29,* 449–456.

Gallup, G. H. (1992, December 10). Remarks presented at the "Too Young to Die" Conference on the National Suicide Survey conducted by Empire Blue Cross and Blue Shield and the Gallup Organization, Inc., New York.

Grabbe, L., Demi, A., Camann, M. A., & Potter, L. (1997). The health status of elderly persons in the last year of life: A comparison of deaths by suicide, injury, and natural causes. *American Journal of Public Health, 87,* 434–437.

Häfner, H. (1997). Special issue on late-onset schizophrenia and the delusional disorder in old age. *European Archives of Psychiatry and Clinical Neuroscience, 247,* 173–218.

Hamilton, M. (1960). A rating scale for depression. *Journal of Neurology, Neurosurgery and Psychiatry, 23,* 56–62.

Hemmelgarn, B., Suissa, S., Huang, A., Boivin, J. F., & Pinard, G. (1997). Benzodiazepine use and the risk of motor vehicle crash in the elderly. *Journal of the American Medical Association, 278,* 27–31.

Heston, L. L., White, J. A., & Mastri, A. R. (1987). Pick's disease: Clinical genetics and natural history. *Archives of General Psychiatry, 4,* 409–411.

Horton-Deutsch, S. L., Clark, D. C., & Farran, C. J. (1992). Chronic dyspnea and suicide in elderly men. *Hospital and Community Psychiatry, 43,* 1198–1203.

Jeste, D. V., Symonds, L. L., & Harris, M. J. (1997). Non-dementia, non-praecox, dementia praecox: Late onset schizophrenia. *American Journal of Geriatric Psychiatry, 5,* 302–317.

Karasu, T. B., Docherty, J. P., & Gelenberg, A. (1993). Practice guidelines for major depressive disorder in adults. *American Journal of Psychiatry, 150*(4), 1–26.

Katz, I. R. (1996). On the inseparability of mental and physical health in aged persons. *American Journal of Geriatric Psychiatry, 4,* 1–16.

Katzman, R. (1986). Alzheimer's disease. *New England Journal of Medicine, 314,* 964–973.

Kelman, H. R., & Thomas, C. (1990). Transitions between community and nursing home residence in an urban elderly population. *Journal of Community Health, 15,* 105–122.

Kennedy, G. J., Kelman, H. R., & Thomas, C. (1991). Persistence and remission of depressive symptoms in late life. *American Journal of Psychiatry, 148,* 174–178.

Kennedy, G. J., Kelman, H. R., Thomas, C., Wisniewski, W., Metz, H., & Bijur, P. (1989). Hierarchy of characteristics associated with depressive symptoms in an urban elderly sample. *American Journal of Psychiatry, 146,* 220–225.

Kennedy, G. J., Metz, H., & Lowinger, R. (1996). Epidemiology and inferences regarding the etiology of late-life suicide. In G. J. Kennedy (Ed.), *Suicide and depression in late life* (pp. 3–22). New York: Wiley.

Kermis, M. D. (1986). The epidemiology of mental disorders in the elderly: A response to the Senate/AARP report. *Gerontologist, 26,* 482–487.

Kohn, R., Westlake, R. J., Rasmussen, M. D., Marsland, R. T., & Norman, W. H. (1997). Clinical features of obsessive-compulsive disorder in elderly patients. *American Journal of Geriatric Psychiatry, 5,* 211–215.

Kusher, M. G., Sher, K. J., & Beitman, B. D. (1990). The relation between alcohol problems and the anxiety disorders. *American Journal of Psychiatry, 147,* 685–689.

Lebowitz, B. D., Pearson, J. L., Schneider, L. S., Reynolds, C. F., Alexopoulos, G. S., Bruce, M. L., Conwell, Y., Katz, I. R., Meyers, B. S., Morrison, M. F., Mossey, J., Niederehe, G., & Parmalee, P. (1997). Diagnosis and treatment of depression in late life: Consensus statement update. *Journal of the American Medical Association, 278,* 1186–1190.

Lilienfeld, D. E., & Perl, D. P. (1994). Projected neurodegenerative disease mortality among minorities in the United States, 1990–2040. *Neuroepidemiology, 13*(4), 179–186.

Madden, J. J., Luhan, J. A., Kaplan, L. A., & Manfredi, H. M. (1952). Non-dementia psychoses in older persons. *Journal of the American Medical Association, 150,* 1567–1570.

Mahendra, B. (1985). Depression and dementia: The multi-faceted relationship. *Psychological Medicine, 15,* 227–236.

Mann, J. J., & Stoff, D. M..(1997). A synthesis of current findings regarding neurobiological correlates and treatment of suicidal behavior. *New York Academy of Science, 836,* 352–363.

Marzuk, P. M., Leon, A. C., Tardiff, K., Morgan, E. B., Marina, S., & Mann J. (1992). The effect of access to lethal methods of injury on suicide rates. *Archives of General Psychiatry, 19,* 451–458.

McDonald, W. M., Krishnan, K. R., Doraiswamy, P. M., & Blazer, D. G. (1996). The occurrence of subcortical hyperintensities in patients with mania. *Psychiatry Research, 40,* 211–220.

McKeith, L. G., Galasko, D., & Kosaka, K. (1996). Consensus guidelines for the clinical and pathologic diagnosis of dementia with Lewy bodies (DLB): Report of the consortium on DLB international workshop. *Neurology, 47,* 1113–1124.

Meehan, P. J., Saltzberg, L. E., & Sattin, R. W. (1991). Suicides among older United States residents: Epidemiologic characteristics and trends. *American Journal of Public Health, 81,* 1198–1200.

Miller, M. (1978). Geriatric suicide: The Arizona study. *Gerontologist, 18,* 488–495.

Mohs, R. C., Breitner, J. C. S., Silverman, J. M., & Davis, K. L. (1987). Alzheimer's disease: Morbid risk among first-degree relatives approximates 50% by 90 years of age. *Archives of General Psychiatry, 44,* 405–408.

Myers, J. K., Weissman, M. M., Tischler, G. L., Holzer, C. E., Leat, P. J., Orvaschel, H., Anthony, J. C., Boyd, J. H., Burke, J. D., Kramer, M., & Stoltzman, R. (1984). Six month prevalence of psychiatric disorders in the community. *Archives of General Psychiatry, 41,* 959–967.

Parikh, R. M., Lipsey, J. R., & Robinson, R. G. (1987). Two-year longitudinal study of post-stroke mood disorders: Dynamic changes in correlates of depression at one and two years. *Stroke, 18,* 579–584.

Peterson, R., Smith, G., & Waring, S. (1999). Mild cognitive impairment: Clinical characterization and outcome. *Archives of Neurology, 56,* 303–308.

Public Health Service. (2001). *National Strategy for Suicide Prevention: Goals and Objectives for Action.* Rockville, MD: U.S. Department of Health and Human Services.

Richards, M., Touchon, J., Ledesert, B., & Richie, K. (1999). Cognitive decline in aging: Are AAMI and AACD distinct entities? *International Journal of Geriatric Psychiatry, 14,* 534–540.

Rovner, B. W., Broadhead, J., Spencer, M., Carson, K., & Folstein, M. F. (1989). Depression and Alzheimer's disease. *American Journal of Psychiatry, 146,* 350–353.

Rovner, B. W., et al. (1990). The prevalence and management of dementia and other psychiatric disorders in the nursing home. *International Psychogeriatrics, 2,* 13–24.

Schultz, S. K., Castillo, C. S., Kosier, J. T., & Robinson, R. G. (1997). Generalized anxiety in depression: Assessment over 2 years after stroke. *American Journal of Geriatric Psychiatry, 5,* 229–237.

Sheikh, J. I., King, R. I., & Taylor, C. B. (1991). Comparative phenomenology of early-onset versus late-onset panic attacks: A pilot study. *American Journal of Psychiatry, 148,* 1231–1233.

Small, G. W., Rabins, P. V., Barry, P. P., Buckholtz, N. S., Dekosky, S. T., Ferris, S. H., Finkel, S. I., Gwyther, L. P., Khachaturian, Z. S., Lebowitz, B. D., McRae, T. D., Morris, J. C., Oakely, R., Schneider, L. S., Streim, J. E., Sunderland, T., Teri, L., & Tune, T. (1997). Diagnosis and treatment of Alzheimer's disease and related disorders. *Journal of the American Medical Association, 278,* 1363–1371.

Smith, S. L., Sherrill, K. A., & Colenda, C. C. (1995). Assessing and treating anxiety in elderly persons. *Psychiatric Services, 46,* 36–42.

United States Public Health Service. (1999). *The Surgeon General's call to action to prevent suicide.* Washington, DC: U.S. Department of Health and Human Services.

Weissman, M. R., Klerman, G. L., Markowitz, J. S., & Ouellette, R. (1989). Suicidal ideation and suicide attempts in panic disorder and attacks. *New England Journal of Medicine, 321,* 1209–1214.

Whanger, A. D. (1989). In E. Busse & D. G. Blazer (Eds.), *Inpatient treatment of the older psychiatric patient in geriatric psychiatry* (pp. 593–634). Washington, DC: American Psychiatric Press.

Young, R. C., Moline, M., & Kleyman, F. (1997). Estrogen replacement therapy and late life mania. *American Journal of Geriatric Psychiatry, 5,* 179–181.

Zung, W. W. K. (1985). A self-rating depression scale. *Archives of General Psychiatry, 12,* 63–70.

# 10

# Counseling Older People and Their Families

## Lynn M. Tepper

Whatever one's age, one has had to witness many transitions in life that are influenced by age, biological changes, social pressures, and family relationships—all part of normal human development from infancy to childhood, adolescence, young adulthood, and older adulthood. During each life transition, it is common for all of us to examine or re-examine our choices, goals, mates, lifestyles, where we live, and so on. Erikson (1963) was the first to acknowledge the fact that we pass from one developmental "crisis" to another, from the time we are infants to the time we become very old. These are certainly punctuation marks along the life span, all requiring some level of examination, or re-examination. Transitions are seldom easy, and may require mental health intervention along the way.

Old age is the life stage with the greatest number of profound crises (Butler, Lewis, & Sunderland, 1998). It is clear that each role transition, with or without a sense of loss, can become a challenge for older persons. As in earlier stages, adaptation to new conditions and situations can bring about a need for support. The older person very often has fewer informal supports such as relatives and friends than younger adults have. Even when family members are abundant, they might not realize that changing circumstances may necessitate intervention.

## ATTITUDES TOWARD SEEKING HELP

Previous generations of older people differ from today's elderly in many ways, many of which have been discussed in other chapters. To add to this ongoing list of differences, the "new old" are more inclined to view mental health as part of their total health picture than have previous generations (Tepper, 1993). However, this group has come a long way in changing its views about mental health services, and some still find mental health concerns difficult to address. The oldest of today's elderly grew up in times when only the most severely mentally ill had psychiatric help, including being remanded to state psychiatric hospitals where conditions were often reprehensible, disgraceful, and truly feared. The future old are more educated, have been exposed to pop psychology in the media (Dr. Brothers, Dr. Ruth, and Dr. Phil), and the explosion of self-help books flooding the market. The combination of factors— increased longevity, their more complex psychosocial and medical conditions, their increased numbers, and their recognition of the importance of mental health services—leads us to believe that there are and will continue to be unprecedented demands on all segments of the mental health community.

## COUNSELING VERSUS PSYCHOTHERAPY

It is important to differentiate between counseling and psychotherapy. Helping to resolve situational problems, many of which are part of normal aging and life changes, is the general goal of counseling. Treating psychopathology or specific mental illness, which may often be related to earlier life experience, is the goal of psychotherapy. Counselors very often assist in revising situational problems rather than reforming and restructuring personalities. They are often more concerned with the here and now, improving life as it now presents itself, than with spending many years in an attempt to look for the root cause of mental health problems of later life. For the purpose of this chapter, counseling and therapy will be used interchangeably. However, psychotherapy, when addressed, will reflect the above definition.

## THE MENTAL HEALTH COMMUNITY: WHO IS THE HELPER?

Today's mental health practice has expanded to include professionals from a wide variety of disciplines and perspectives. Although their titles, degrees, and training may vary, they share the common goal of improving quality of life. Psychiatrists, medical doctors who specialize in psychiatric disorders, represent the medical model of treatment, most often using a combination of psychotherapy and medication to attain a desirable mental health goal. Psychologists, with doctorates in psychology, provide counseling and psychotherapy with a wide range of techniques designed to meet the specific needs of their patients. They rely on "talk therapy," as they are unable to prescribe medication to change behavior. Both psychiatrists and psychologists work in hospitals, private practice, community health centers, and nursing homes. However, clinical social workers provide the majority of mental health care to persons of all ages, especially to older people. They work in all of the above settings and use both counseling and psychotherapy to achieve their goals. If they are properly licensed, all of these practitioners are eligible to receive reimbursement from private insurance companies, Medicare, and Medicaid. The nursing profession, especially geriatric nurses and nurse practitioners, provide increasing amounts of mental health services to older people, as do psychiatric nurses. Counselors trained in psychology and counseling at the graduate level work in a variety of settings, including mental health centers and private practice. Counselors with less training also can be found in government sponsored agencies for the aging, community mental health centers, and family counseling centers in the community. Some may also use alternative therapeutic approaches, such as pet-facilitative therapy or environmental change therapies. There are also increasing numbers of occupational therapists who use mental health interventions to improve life quality for their patients while improving physical functioning. Recreation therapists use a variety of individual and group approaches, with therapeutic activity modalities for elders who are isolated, depressed, or cognitively impaired. Among all of the above fields, specialized training in gerontology and geriatrics has increased in the past twenty years, but not nearly enough practitioners have been trained to meet the rising needs.

## MENTAL HEALTH GOALS

Social workers, psychologists, nurses, administrators, physicians, physical therapists, occupational therapists, clergy, lawyers, recreation workers, and planners of programs for older persons all share the common goal of improving the quality of life for their clients and patients, and often become involved in the lives of individuals and their families. Solving problems related to daily living is a goal for many who provide services to the elderly. As with younger adults, many of the situations requiring counseling are crisis oriented and situational, demanding relatively quick intervention. Other problems requiring counseling are developmental and may not require long-term psychotherapy with the goal of fundamental personality change. Some problems will have no appropriate or satisfactory solutions. The emotional pain that almost always accompanies the illness or death of a spouse or loved one, the psychological dislocation associated with retirement, terminal illness, chronic pain, loneliness, social role changes and losses, and financial maintenance problems are prominent in the lives of older persons. Counseling may address concerns that are the direct result of these situational changes. These concerns may present as feelings of depression, inadequacy, poor self-concept, discouragement, paralysis of will (intense lack of motivation), unrealistic expectations, and feelings of alienation.

Much of the research on middle age and old age has supported the notion that personality organization and coping style are major factors in predicting successful adaptation to growing old. Aging is generally not the sole reason for maladaptive behavior. Coping styles developed in childhood and adolescence and reinforced in earlier adulthood are usually still present in the older person. Consequently, establishing counseling goals can be very challenging but extremely worthwhile. The good news is that there is potential for change that can lead to greater self-acceptance, the ability to reduce and control anxiety, increased self-esteem, a renewed sense of empowerment, and the ability to come to terms with life as it has been and is being lived.

Herr and Weakland (1979) have identified the existence of several restrictions when counseling older people. The lack of time for counseling may be a limitation, especially when a service provider's job may not include time for counseling per se. Another time restriction may be the client's time. Years of psychotherapy may not be feasible when someone is very old and in need of more immediate solutions to situational problems. Another limitation may be the lack of an appropriate place to talk. This may be a problem in settings such as senior centers, care facilities, or on home visits. Finding a location that is private, comfortable, and accessible to the older person can be a challenge. Economic limitations may also be a factor, as a large segment of this population is living on a fixed income, with little access to health insurance other than Medicare or Medicaid. The stigma that some of this generation still associates with mental health intervention can also be a limitation. These attitudes are changing, and the elderly cohort of the twenty-first century is already viewing counseling and psychotherapy as a more acceptable part of its total health care needs (Tepper, 1993).

## THE AGING FAMILY: THERAPEUTIC INTERVENTION

In consideration of the stage-wise development of families throughout the life span, it is often acknowledged that the older person is usually at the stage in which the family has ceased expanding, and beginning to contract in size. The author has all too often observed that when this age group is discussed in professional literature, they are often stereotypically described as individuals with little or no relationship to families. However, in reality, the older person's family often has expanded to include their adult children and their spouses, and their grandchildren and great-grandchildren. Even the family therapy literature has largely overlooked the relationship between older people and their families (Gutheil & Tepper, 1994). Anderson (1988) has observed that family therapists have had little to say about older people, relegating them to the role of filling spaces in genograms in order to clarify the problems of younger generations. Viewing the older person in primarily individual terms has resulted in insufficient attention paid to the important interrelationships between older people and their families.

One of the myths about the aged is that they are abandoned by their families and deposited into nursing homes when they require care. In point of fact, only 5% of those 65 and older are in nursing homes. This small number is even smaller when we consider that three times this number (15%) is actually in need of care. When we examine the statistics, it is easy to see that as a society we are doing twice as much family caregiving as we are thought to be doing. Older people are very much part of families, whether married, widowed, or never married.

As life expectancy increases, so do the number of generations in a family. Many older people are part of four- or five-generation families. Longer life expectancy, coupled with people having fewer children, has resulted in the average person spending more time with aging parents than as a parent of a child under 18 years of age (Bengston, Rosenthal, & Burton, 1990).

Society has always tended to view older people in terms of their potential as burdens to their adult children, but a more balanced view has recently emerged (Gutheil & Tepper, 1994). As was discussed in chapters 1 and 2, increased life expectancy and improved health status have resulted in a new definition of older people. Research has shown that older people frequently are supportive to their families, especially to those who are coping with stressful life events (Greenberg & Becker, 1988). They are often as important in family counseling as their family can be for counseling them. Counseling older families requires special skills, many of which are rooted in family therapy. Herr and Weakland (1979) have recommended the following guidelines for counseling elders in a family context:

1. *Set realistic goals.* Addressing situational problems which are immediate, as well as problems which reduce their quality of life should be primary counseling goals. The restructuring of personality and psychoanalytic treatment may be less relevant in later life.

2. *Encourage reluctant families to share problems.* This difficulty in sharing feelings may well explain why the family is having problems in the first place. It is helpful for the counselor to reframe the approach so that it becomes clear that the family is assisting the counselor if they tell him or her about the problem.

3. *Assist families in defining the problem.* Families often have difficulty in defining the real problem. This is especially true when the problem is perceived to be caused by the individual, not the family. Families may be defensive when faced with the idea that family interaction (or lack of interaction) may contribute to problematic behavior. Without clear definitions, there are no solutions.

4. *Gain full participation of the family.* This is usually more easily said than done. Hesitant participants need gentle encouragement. If all family members are not available for counseling, several are usually sufficient to communicate the effects of family interaction and to discuss possible resolutions.

5. *Deal with family anger.* Sometimes feelings of helplessness and frustration can manifest as the family's "attacking" the counselor, perhaps in challenging competence or experience. Honesty and validation of the underlying feelings is the best approach; defensiveness will lead to disaster!

6. *Determine what the older person's family has been doing about the problem.* Question as to what has proven to be successful and unsuccessful, and why. This is often a good place to start brainstorming new approaches.

7. *Make sense of the family system.* This involves taking the time to step back and digest all that has been learned about how the family operates. It requires examining the various facets of the problem, analyzing the context in which family communication takes place, identifying family roles such as who displays emotions and who gets the last word, deciding who the identified client is, and considering the expression of personal power of each family member and how it may contribute to alliances within the family unit.

8. *Express empathy, but reserve judgment.* The expression of approval or disapproval is not necessary to validate how family members feel or what they do.

9. *Mobilize the energy of the family.* Assisting the family to move forward toward a solution may or may not necessitate further counselor interventions. If the family has difficulty moving forward, the task is to lead them gently around the obstacles that are holding them back.

Family counseling can also be helpful for families of institutionalized persons. It can help them deal with the feelings, stresses, and pressures they may be experiencing about their older relative. Groups organized for this purpose can also provide members with knowledge about Alzheimer's disease, depression, medication usage, physical changes, the meaning of institutional life, and guidelines for visitation (Weiner, Brok, & Snadowsky, 1987).

### The Case of Libby F.

*Libby F. is a 88-year-old widow with limited mobility but full mental capacity. Her husband passed away several months ago, leaving her alone in their Florida retirement house, for the first time in their more than 60 years of marriage. Libby's adult children, now with their own adult children, grandchildren, and professions, live in a northern metropolitan city. They discussed the possibility of her moving back north to be near her family, which would also make it easier for them to keep an eye on their mother. They seriously considered some of the local older adult living alternatives discussed in chapter 3. However, after returning to Florida, Libby shortly discovered a large circle of friends and neighbors, most of them widows themselves, who befriended her. She bonded with these women, who became a second family to her, often helping her with activities that required mobility, such as shopping. Needless to say, plans for moving up north were abandoned . . . at least for now!*

Making a dramatic change in living arrangements shortly after becoming widowed is not usually advisable. The older person's input is primary when important decisions like this one are being made.

## DEMENTIA AND THE FAMILY

When reversible conditions are ruled out, and senile dementia becomes the primary diagnosis, the family often finds it difficult to mobilize forces for the purpose of caregiving. Two issues are central and need to be explored: (1) How can a family cope with the frustrating, embarrassing, and often disruptive behavior of a person with dementia? and (2) How can the caregiver find ways to ease the stress and help the loved one? The author has observed that the amount of burden family members experience caring for a person with dementia is related to the support they receive from other family members and friends. In many cases, the primary caregiver benefits from individual or group counseling at first. But without involvement of other family members in the form of more support to the primary caregiver, individual counseling is often not the answer.

Regular family meetings that address the tensions and imbalances in the family system created by the patient's disabilities can be a helpful intervention. As impairments increase, there is additional pressure on others in the family to take over tasks. These tasks are not only instrumental, like managing money or cooking, but also affective, like providing empathetic contact or being a confidante. Families benefit greatly from meeting regularly, either with or without the services of a therapist. They need to assess the changes taking place in the family because of the responsibilities of the primary caregiver, and to identify ways of compensating that can keep the family functioning as a cohesive unit.

Primary care functions have usually been divided along sex lines, with women bearing most of the hands-on responsibilities, and men providing most of the emotional and/or financial support. With the current shifts in family structure as a result of the increasing numbers of women in the work force, this is changing. More formal (paid) caregiving may be done by hired individuals or institutional placement may be sought.

The question often arises: Who will do the caregiving? Most often it is the spouse. A myth persists that we as a society toss our relatives into nursing homes. On the contrary. Only a minority of mentally compromised or physically frail elderly are placed into institutions; a majority are taken care of at home. But when families do elect to care for a loved one at home, there are a number of critical issues that should be addressed by the family caregivers: (1) When the problems caused by the dementia are raised, does the family tend to get off the subject? (2) Are some family members' opinions given more credence than others? (3) What was the previous role that the patient played in the family system before the illness? (4) What is the caregiver's role in this system? (5) Is the caregiver powerful or viewed as inadequate by other family members? (6) Are there longstanding family problems or conflicts that impact on caregiving?

Social issues must also be addressed by families. The most common concerns expressed by family caregivers include reports that friends have stopped calling; feeling cut off from the community; feeling isolated from the world; feeling conflicted about needs to establish relationships, perhaps intimate ones; wondering how to deal with these decisions; concern about the probability of also being afflicted with Alzheimer's disease or dementia; and wondering who the true victim of the disease is . . . the patient or the caregiver.

Support groups for caregivers have increased in number, and have been found to be highly effective for reducing stress. They are now available in a majority of communities and offer many benefits, especially in that they allow caregivers to share information with one another and to assist members to better understand their own experiences. Support groups ideally should be offered together with a multifaceted program, as some people will do better with one-to-one counseling, and others with a combination of both support groups and one-to-one counseling. Stress-management programs to assist caregivers in restructuring or modifying their lifestyles to promote stress-reduction activities are often offered in the community by adult education programs, or courses at local colleges and community health centers (Tepper, 1993).

## GROUP THERAPY IN LATER LIFE

The use of group therapy with older people is worthwhile, both in the community and in institutions. Yalom (1985), a pioneer in group approaches, described ten benefits of group therapy: (1) imparting information, (2) instillation of hope, (3) universality (problems in common), (4) altruism, (5) corrective recapitulation (re-think and change attitudes about) of the primary family group, (6) development of socializing techniques, (7) imitative behavior, (8) interpersonal behavior, (9) group cohesiveness, and (10) catharsis. Community programs, including senior centers, day care centers, and other senior citizens' programs use group work, with the goals of personal growth, emotional satisfaction, and positive social experiences for participants. Specialized groups are organized for specific purposes, such as groups for widows, the recently bereaved, those with demanding caregiving responsibilities, couples therapy, and older people with various health problems who share common concerns. Leadership of these groups may be active or passive, and may include teaching, protecting, explaining, questioning, confronting, and reassuring (Butler et al., 1998).

Group therapy for those in institutions such as homes for the aged can also benefit significantly from a variety of mental health interventions (Tepper, 1993). Just living in an institution is likely to affect a resident's mental health; apathy, lack of initiative, resentment, and loss of interest in life can affect their emotional status. Mentally impaired elders can also benefit from group therapy to help reduce behavioral problems and even renew interest in their surroundings (Butler et al., 1998). Examples of group themes are reality orientation, which will accustom them to their environment; sensory training, to rekindle their sensory, verbal, movement, and intellectual abilities; pet therapy, to promote social interaction and enhance self-esteem and a sense of control; reminiscence groups, which can be useful in exploring fond memories and coming to terms with their lives; and remotivation groups, to reawaken previous elements of their personality, and lead them to take an interest in their surroundings (Tepper, 1993).

## LIFE REVIEW: THE THERAPEUTIC USE OF REMINISCENCE

The concept of life review has been part of the literature and practice of gerontology, psychology, psychiatry, social work, and nursing for the past thirty years. It was first developed by Lewis and Butler in 1974, to assist older people to use past experience to assist with both memory and life satisfaction (Lewis & Butler, 1974). This approach involves taking an extensive autobiography from the client and other family members in order to put together a summation of one's life work, reexamine one's life, overcome guilt, reconcile family relationships, and resolve personal conflicts (Butler et al., 1998).

There are many ways to accomplish this. It is helpful to gather family photo albums, scrapbooks, and other memorabilia, and even make a trip back to the "old neighborhood" and other places of importance to assist with this process. Putting together a family tree also helps, as it renews old memories and results in a finished product which can be passed on to grandchildren. This adds another goal to life review, that of achieving generativity, transmitting knowledge and values to future generations, thus adding prestige to being the oldest in a family. The finding of one's cultural and ethnic roots has become popular over recent years, and ethnic pride is a rewarding outcome for all those involved.

Lieberman and Tobin (1983) have confirmed that reminiscence is a crucial part of the emotional livelihood of an older person, helping to resolve past conflicts and enabling the development of a coherent life history. Reevaluating one's life, coming to terms with life as one has lived it, is also important for facing death. This has been acknowledged in the gerontological literature to the present day as an important modality in counseling and psychotherapy with older adults. Reminiscence and life review can be accomplished individually and in groups and in a variety of settings. These include but are not limited to senior centers, nursing homes, adult residences, and community health settings. Groups can be led by a variety of mental health professionals and can provide socialization as well as therapy.

## CONCLUSION

Although the focus of this chapter is on counseling and therapy for older people with typical maladjustment problems, the issues and strategies presented here are not intended for those with severe psychiatric problems or severe psychopathology. Efforts for counseling older people are most widely used when sadness, lack of initiative, inadequacy, unrealistic goals, low self-esteem, discouragement, and lack of a sense of belonging begin to interfere with their quality and enjoyment of life. The developmental issues that most commonly confront people in later life, such as loss of relatives, friends, job, prestige, health; a supportive environment; and social status, can be the focus of counseling and therapeutic interventions with this group.

Older people usually do not want to be dependent on others any more than other age groups welcome dependency (Tepper, 1994). They want to preserve every bit of independence, personal autonomy, and self-respect. Providing counseling services to people with such values and attitudes is not easy, but it is extremely rewarding.

## REFERENCES

Anderson, D. (1988). The quest for a meaningful old age. *Family Therapy Networker, 12*(4), 17–22, 72–25.

Bengston, V., Rosenthal, C., & Burton, B. (1990). Families and aging: Diversity and heterogeneity. In R. H. Binstock & L. K. George (Eds.), *Handbook of aging and the social sciences* (pp. 19–44). San Diego: Academic Press.

Butler, R. N., Lewis, M., & Sunderland, T. (1998). Psychotherapy and environmental therapy. *Aging and mental health* (pp. 346–375). Boston: Allyn & Bacon.

Erikson, E. H. (1963). *Childhood and society* (2nd ed.). New York: Norton.

Greenberg, J. S., & Becker, M. (1988). Aging parents as family resources. *Gerontologist, 28*, 786–791.

Gutheil, I., & Tepper, L. M. (1994). The aging family: Ethnic and cultural considerations. In E. P. Congress (Ed.), *Multicultural perspectives in working with families* (pp 89–108). New York: Springer.

Herr, J. J., & Weakland, J. H. (1979). *Counseling elders and their families.* New York: Springer.

Lewis, M. I., & Butler, R. N. (1974). Life review therapy: Putting memories to work in group and individual therapy. *Geriatrics, 29,* 165–169.

Lieberman, M. A., & Tobin, S. S. (1983). *The experience of old age: Stress, coping and survival.* New York: Basic Books.

Tepper, L. M. (1993). Group therapy with the elderly. In L. M. Tepper & J. A. Toner (Eds.), *Long term care* (pp. 136–146). Philadelphia: Charles.

Tepper, L. M. (1994). Developmental theories in the second half of life. In I. Gutheil (Ed.), *Work with older people* (pp. 29–41). New York: Fordham University Press.

Weiner, M. B., Brok, A. J., & Snadowsky, A. M. (1987). *Working with the aged: Practical approaches in the institution and in the community* (2nd ed.). Norwalk, CT: Appleton-Century-Crofts.

Yalom, I. D. (1985). *The theory and practice of group psychotherapy* (3rd ed.). New York: Basic Books.

# 11

# End-of-Life Issues from a Social Service Perspective

## Sally S. Robinson and Lynn M. Tepper

This chapter introduces a social service perspective in which collaborative helping strategies promote the delivery of assistance that humanizes and brings coherence to the end-of-life journey of elders and their loved ones. It begins with a discussion of the major factors within social service that are most effective in understanding and intervening in the end-of-life concerns and circumstances of older adults and their families.

Specific end-of-life social service responses are generally offered to (1) elders 85+ who have not been medically diagnosed as terminally ill, but who are facing, together with their caregivers, increasing loss of function due to chronic illnesses such as Chronic Obstructive Pulmonary Disease (COPD) or Congestive Heart Failure (CHF), or degenerative diseases like Alzheimer's disease, and may be aware of a compressed future; (2) the oldest old, who may not be suffering from chronic diseases, but are nevertheless frail and need assistance with their activities of daily living, and who are also aware of a compressed future; and (3) hospice patients and their families who are facing patients' imminent death.

Interventions discussed will include both interdisciplinary and multidisciplinary approaches to service and social work with families of the above identified elders. Special attention will be paid to the stressors common to end-of-life caregivers, both family and professional. The grief of elders and their families and friends who are mourning personal losses associated with imminent demise or other progressive loss of functionality will be discussed along with the bereavement issues that survivors face. A social service perspective for intervention with Alzheimer's patients and their families will also be presented.

185

## AN INCLUSIVE SOCIAL PERSPECTIVE

The word "social" is used here to distinguish the care being described from that of the skilled medical care of a physician or nurse. Here, social care means all types of social services such as individual casework, care/case management, assisted referrals for concrete community services, custodial assistance with the activities of daily life, supportive individual and group counseling, and psychotherapeutic interventions in life adjustment problems and mood disorders.

True to the multidisciplinary focus of this book, a social service perspective for understanding and addressing end-of-life issues must be informed by and encompass the other perspectives of aging.

## DEMOGRAPHY AND HEALTH STATUS

A useful social service perspective is shaped by public health considerations which, in turn, are influenced by current aging demographics and population trends. In order to understand and predict the availability of social care resources for end-of-life needs, the social worker must be aware of the current and projected size of this population and know whether more or fewer of these elderly are, or will be facing, imminent end of life or protracted dying in an existence characterized by chronic illness requiring ongoing social care associated with their medical condition. The social worker must also be informed about the extent to which the current and projected oldest-old, those 85 and over, are relatively free of disease, but are experiencing progressive frailty. Assisting an individual client with life adjustment (in the form of counseling) or concrete service needs (in the form of actual services, such as meals, medical intervention, and housing) is more or less effective depending upon the client's health status and the health care resources available. Further, an individual's access to needed health care at any point of time is associated with the pressure of supply and demand for health care, degree of social necessity to conserve health care resources.

A note about the caseworker's role: so-called micro social work does not preclude a worker from assessing the elder's place in the current and future contexts of health status and care needs and, then, accordingly, from becoming appropriately involved in professional advocacy for helping resources. It is the writers' view that to be relevant, social policy must utilize experiential knowledge gained in service. It is part of a responsible social service perspective to use that knowledge for informed advocacy. With regard to both current and future end-of-life service populations, the demographics discussed in chapter 1 are extremely pertinent to service providers, especially the tremendous growth of the oldest-old. During the period between 1990 and 2000, the entire subset of persons 85+ increased by 38% and the centenarians within that group increased by 35%. The subset of elders 75–84 increased by 23% (Smith & Hetzel, 2000). The rapid growth of this oldest of the old among the total 65+ population and the projected concomitant increase of Alzheimer's disease alert us to the probable accompanying increase of elders and their families facing end-of-life concerns. The social worker should be alert to the public health impact of these elderly: Are the required medical and other care resources available, and will they be available to the future elderly? (Ahronheim, 1997; Centers for Disease Control, 2003; Rea, Popeski, & Zinchiak, 2001). Social service interventions may be limited by lack of medical and concrete services. For example, without freedom from pain, or without the functional independence or help to procure and prepare food, social work to ameliorate emotional problems is impossible. An effective social work perspective should include a thorough awareness of health initiatives in place by both private organizations and government to address this population's growing needs. This must include strategies to promote wellness, thereby pushing back the age at which end-of-life needs become necessary, with accompanying demand for formal service provision (U.S. Department of HHS, 2001).

## ECONOMIC FACTORS: WHO PAYS FOR WHAT?

Whether any given social service intervention is primarily macro (planning and administration) or micro (case management or counseling), a useful social service perspective must be influenced by economic factors. Who is paying for what? How does the payer impact the social services available to a particular individual or to a class of elders facing end-of-life service needs? A social worker's ability to help will be curtailed or enhanced by the economic context of service. It will also be influenced by public sanction, or lack of public sanction, for applying tax dollars to end-of-life health and social services (Austin & Fleisher, 2003; Buntin & Huskamp, 2002). Chapter 12, "Financing Health Care," will provide more details on health insurance benefits and limitations. The availability of social services is actually most typically benefit-driven. Although private-pay providers do exist, these are not yet affordable for a majority of older people (a subsequent section will discuss this option in more detail). Therefore, a practical social service perspective must be realistic as to the kinds and amount of available helping opportunities, without assumptions or presumptions as to the proportionality of these opportunities to assessed need.

## PRIVATE GERIATRIC CARE MANAGERS

Many of the oldest old are geographically separated from family for many reasons, including living in out-of-town retirement communities and remaining in the old neighborhood after adult children have moved away. Adult children may also be busy working and managing their own families, or may choose not to provide the intensity of care required. An alternative to publicly assisted community or institutional programs are "Geriatric Care Managers," private practitioners of end-of-life care, who are available on a fee-for-service basis and usually take on a limited number of private clients. These professionals are mostly licensed social workers and psychologists. They provide in-depth assessment and a personalized care plan for their clients. After linking these elders to services, these care managers continue to regularly oversee the delivery of these services. They can also provide medical, financial, and legal referrals, and ongoing counseling to the elder as well as family members. An effective social service perspective must include an awareness of private care managers.

## RELATIONAL AND TRANSITIONAL IMPLICATIONS OF LEGAL CHOICES

Legal issues play an important part in developing a useful perspective for planning and delivering social services. In the area of relational and transitional end-of-life concerns, legal issues are paramount to the elder who is proactively looking forward to that end stage of life with advance directives and to the elder who is reactively coping with the experience of terminal illness. The reader is urged to study chapter 13 in this volume, "Issues in Elder Law," for particulars regarding the legal aspects of planning for one's death.

End-of-life legal choices can be enormously facilitated by a social service perspective that recognizes the relational and transitional aspects of such choices. Conversely, a perspective that does not include legal decision making as a social concern may hinder the elder's ability to consider his or her legal options in their social context. Decisions regarding advance directives may alter relationships of the elder who is facing imminent death and also of the elder who may not be terminally ill, but has made legal choices, acknowledging the reality of a compressed future. Naming a health care proxy or other delegation of authority may not only reflect in whom an elder's trust is placed, but with whom his or her trust is *not* placed. This may result in hurt feelings and even in court cases where plaintiffs argue that trust has been misplaced. The social worker may be called upon to mediate among an elder's family and friends who are not on the same page regarding the elder's end-of-life legal choices. Other relational issues may be revealed in an elder's end-of-life legal decision making, especially in those choices that involve the personal autonomy and control of everyone involved.

### Case Study

*Megan Quigley, a social worker-bereavement counselor at Kershaw County Medical Center in South Carolina, relates the story of a 93-year-old male hospice patient with congestive heart failure, whose autonomy and self-efficacy were threatened and indeed abrogated when he made a gift of his house to his daughter and son-in-law. These family members resided with him in the house and were his primary caregivers. Megan relates that the dying man transferred ownership of his house because he felt that the burden of his care would be thereby lessened for his daughter and son-in-law. Whether or not their sense of burden was reduced by her father's legal choice, the daughter's actions and those of her husband became preemptive and independent of the elder's stated wishes. She hovered over her father, feeling that even leaving his bed would put him at undue risk. His activities—already curtailed by his illness—were further reduced and he strongly and realistically felt a loss of control and personhood to the extent that he refused to participate in holidays that were previously times of meaning and happiness for him. "I am not in Christmas this year" he said.*

In this case, the legal "remedy" made in a social context of wishing to be cared for without rancor or resentment, resulted in an assault on the elder's sense of self and relational shifting with his loved ones. Clearly, his legal decision making in this case would have benefited from some pre-choice counseling. The client's daughter and son-in-law might have benefitted as well from counseling with respect to issues of control: feelings of helplessness to prevent client's imminent demise, father's need to retain personal autonomy, and their need to protect the father by controlling his process of dying. Certainly, the social worker was needed post-choice.

Transitional issues also may require a social service response. Perhaps the most common end of life transitional issue is the change from so-called curative care to palliative comfort care, in which an acknowledgment is made of imminent death (Parry, 1989). Helping older people and their families make the transition from expecting cure to accepting the end of life is a multidisciplinary effort involving medical and other care providers. However, *change* is the special province of social service providers. This change, from embracing life to meeting death, is perhaps the greatest change a person ever faces. Although death is part of everyone's life, experiencing one's own imminent death as a stage of life is fraught with difficulty, if not contradiction of immense proportion. Whereas death denotes the actual end of life, end of life really denotes the period of time, days, weeks, or months during which one is alive but moving toward death. Hence, end of life is a dynamic concept, often viewed as a stage either physically due to terminal illness, or psychologically due to progressive reduction of functionality that is not related directly to illness, such as sensory and mobility losses. An elder convalescing from hospitalization for acute illness may view recovery more as delayed mortality than cure. It has been this (S. R.) author's experience that the meaning of mortality changes for many convalescing elderly to an eventuality—something that may have been successfully avoided "this time," but definitely part of the foreseeable future. This state of mind represents a major psychological transition which, although assisted by legal remedies/decisions discussed in this book, often is helped equally by the empathic, person-centered counseling of a social worker or other mental health professional. For psychotherapeutic interventions for older people and their families, please pay special attention to Chapter 10, "Counseling Older People and their Families."

## DIFFERENTIATION OF END-OF-LIFE TRANSITIONS

A social service perspective that includes transitions as a major part of the end-of-life process is an almost prima facie requirement for service to ill older people. However, there is another subset of older people who typically may not experience acute or even chronic illness as a prelude to acknowledgment of the end of life. This group of elderly, most notably those 85 and over, may be relatively free of diseases, but they (or others) measure their futures in terms of the reduction of the number of activities of daily life they can perform independently. Rather than experiencing end of life as a phenomenon of disease requiring the transitions discussed above, these elders may be described as "squaring the curve." Morbidity is not a significant factor in their demise; their physical systems just gradually wind down. When a recently widowed wife of a man who died in his late nineties was asked the cause of her husband's death, she replied that he just "went" in his sleep, that he had no particular new medical problem, but that his body "kind of just gave out." As discussed above, end of life is usually a period of gradual termination of one's life processes due to the progression of one or more illnesses or diseases. In this paradigm, death is basically the outcome of a pathological assault upon the body. Even though the hospice care alternative humanizes this process, it remains a pathological one.

A comprehensive social service perspective should distinguish among the three types of end-of-life stages identified above if service is to be effective and relevant. When Medicare and the Older Americans Act were enacted in 1965, everyone 65 and older was lumped under the term "senior citizen," and viewed as persons with all the same needs and problems. In the decades that followed, aging demographics revealed a different reality. End-of-life issues must not only be classified as to type (legal, economic, relational, transitional), but must be addressed with consideration of the functional and medical status of those experiencing them.

## SOCIAL SERVICE TO NON-HOSPICE POPULATIONS: COST

Although non-hospice elderly face similar end-of-life concerns as those officially diagnosed as terminally ill, social services may not be as readily available to them. Like hospice patients, they are struggling with progressively decreasing functionality. A social service perspective must include an appreciation of the financing mechanisms in place for the delivery of social care services. This will generally enable the differentiated application of non-hospice dollars to help this group, whether through Medicare home health care or other federal and state programs. In order to use these resources on behalf of the non-hospice but frail elderly and their families, a social service end-of-life perspective cannot be limited to hospice patients.

## END-OF-LIFE CONCERNS RELATIVE
## TO ALZHEIMER'S DISEASE

Although Alzheimer's disease is terminal by definition, the rate of degeneration for each person varies along with the symptoms of this disease (Komaroff, 2002). Therefore, patients and their families may face a delayed mortality of several years to more than a decade, depending on the course of the disease and other health factors. Depending upon their cognitive status and/or their families, when do patients begin to address end-of-life issues? This question is crucial for the development of adequate service responses to this disease which is increasing along with the 85+ population. Whereas 10% of persons 65+ have Alzheimer's disease, almost 50% of those 85+ have received this diagnosis (Federal Forum on Aging Related Statistics, 2002). It is probable that others 85 and older have not been diagnosed with Alzheimer's but may be in the first stages of this disease, in which it may not be differentiated easily from other dementias. As this 85+ group is the fastest growing U.S. population, Alzheimer's patients and their families are a burgeoning service group for numerous professional disciplines. It differs from other dementias in that its progression may include an inconsistent and fluctuating array of problems. Though team-based coordination of care, including medical, mental health, and social service expertise, is called for in order to achieve effective interventions, non-institutional opportunities for this kind of assistance are not readily available to patients who are not wealthy enough to pay privately, but are not poor enough to be eligible for Medicaid. To add to this complication, they may not be medically qualified for hospice, with the required 6-months-to-live prognosis. Institutional care is currently the most sought-after living arrangement for Alzheimer's patients in the last stages of the disease, but high quality care centers currently have waiting lists. Moreover, these facilities may become less available as the number of Alzheimer's patients increases. Even now about 75% of persons with Alzheimer's live at home. And, the same amount—75%—of care for them is provided by family and friends (Komaroff, 2002).

Awareness of the social care needs of Alzheimer's patients at the many different stages of the disease is crucial for the effective organization and targeting of services to this group. Again, a social service perspective must be inclusive in order to engender or promote the practical, individualized assistance that Alzheimer's patients and their families need in order to physically, psychologically, and financially cope with this particularly insidious assault on one's physical and mental person. On one hand, the interventions of medical professionals may be constrained by their duties, responsibilities, time limitations, and activities required by health insurers. On the other hand, social work—if part of the insurance package at all—is not as functionally constrained. As a less costly intervention relative to the medical ones, social work is defined more fluidly and, as such, can include amelioration of a range of problems including complex psychosocial issues. The scope and type of intervention described as "social" makes this profession key to any multi-disciplinary team-based service. Although the blurring of roles—typical in teamwork—may be problematic for medical professionals, role flexibility is one of the defining characteristics of social work. Finally, relative to family caregiving to people with Alzheimer's, families may serve as the patient's surrogate for many end-of-life decisions typically faced by elderly who are not cognitively intact. The varying, fluctuating, and inconsistent progression of the disease may make it seem to loved ones as an almost temporary state. Particularly in the early stages of the disease, family members may have difficulty making decisions for the patient. They may even view the illness as transitory when the patient's symptoms seem to disappear from time to time. A social service perspective that includes an appreciation of the physiological progression of the disease is important to help family members adjust their relationship with and their expectations for the patient so as to provide the most sensitive, effective care.

## HOSPICE: COMFORT CARE

America's first hospice began in 1974, providing palliative care in the home. It was not until 1986 that Medicare Hospice benefit was made permanent by Congress. In 1989, the six-months Medicare benefit lifetime limitation was removed, although it remained in place for the physician's admitting diagnosis of terminal illness. By 1993, the number of Medicare Hospices grew by over 400% from 310 in 1984 to 1,288 (Hospice Association of America, 2003).

Whether hospice care is delivered in the home or in an institution, the emphasis is on comforting the patient physically, emotionally, and spiritually during the last months or less of life. Medicare and other health insurance policies may provide for hospice care, including medical services, medications, equipment, nursing, supplies, trained volunteers, and social service to the patient and family before the patient's death and after for 12 months. Key to the hospice program is pain management. When physicians decide that curative treatment will not help, they can then make a diagnosis of terminal illness, usually, but not always, with the patient's and the family's informed consent. Patients and their families may express their desire to follow physicians' orders, but are not interested in knowing the basis for such orders. Palliative care, which manages pain but is not curative, is the primary and essential type of care in a hospice program. But in order to help the patient and family accept the criterion for palliative pain management ("imminent demise"), pain management must be acknowledged as part of a total multidisciplinary program of compassionate and comprehensive palliative care. Palliative care, however, is not limited to the management of physical pain, and should always address psychic pain as well. Spiritual support under a hospice program may be the central part of emotional support. According to an experienced sociologist, also a nun, patients with some past ties to organized religion usually are open to religious intervention, as are their families (Munley, 1983).

## CULTURAL COMPETENCY IN END-OF-LIFE CARE

As the older population grows by leaps and bounds, it is also becoming more ethnically diverse. Older people who have immigrated to the U.S., and even the children of immigrants, have a stronger cultural heritage than succeeding generations will have (Gutheil & Tepper, 1997). Along with ethnic diversity comes a consideration of culture. Sensitivity to the patient's culture must also be a part of an effective hospice program (Burger, 2002). The social worker is central to the cultural and concomitant psychosocial issues that should be addressed by any hospice program. Burger (2002) identified several skills and abilities central to culturally competent care, including:

- The ability to identify cultural differences
- An acceptance by the care provider that cultural differences are important
- An awareness of whether the patient and his or her family practice the particular rites and traditions of their culture with respect to the end-of-life process
- A knowledge of who in the family is culturally acceptable as the primary decision maker for end-of-life care
- A willingness and the necessary skills to question in an open-ended-manner in order to learn about a person's culture and to ensure the provider's understanding of different meanings of the same word in different cultures
- The use of trained interpreters when a language barrier exists

## HOSPICE CARE TEAMWORK

The social work role in hospice care can be a sensitive bridge of understanding between the patient and his or her family that can provide a path of supportive care that flows from patient and family to the entire interdisciplinary hospice care team, including medical professionals and volunteers. The following observations regarding this 'bridge of understanding' are based upon an interview with Megan Quigley, a young licensed social worker working in the home hospice program of a county medical center in South Carolina. She has been practicing social work since 1998, primarily in home settings with home health care and currently with a home hospice program. She stated that the success of any hospice program relies upon multidisciplinary teamwork, where a blurring of roles is not only inevitable but desirable for seamless care. She pointed out that the hospice team of doctor, nurse, social worker, and volunteer constitute a surrogate family for the patient and family caregivers. As such, the hospice team must know and respect each other's individual areas of expertise, but at the same time, pick up from each other a caring theme that permeates each team member's individual function. A physician at a local nursing home supported the above observations and commented that an interdisciplinary approach can only work if each care provider delivers care systematically, with emphasis on constant communication to ensure care that is part of a sequential and collaborative process. Conversely, an undesirable inter-disciplinary approach is a "haphazard assortment of actions and reactions" so that patient care fragments territorially according to the domain interests of the various disciplines involved (Levenson, 2002). In point of fact, multidisciplinary care provision does not assure teamwork. A social work perspective that is not informed by thoughtful analysis of which professional behaviors constitute teamwork and which do not is inadequate for truly collaborative work. The reader is referred to chapters 2, 5, 6, and 10 in this volume regarding the coordination of care for multi-problem elders in need of a number of health and mental health interventions, and chapter 16, which is exclusively de-voted to the theme of teamwork.

## FACING UP TO FEELINGS AT END-OF-LIFE

The hospice social worker interviewed above identified poor communication as common to end-of-life problems in hospice programs. She likened these problems to the "elephant in the room"; everyone knows it's there, but no one wants to acknowledge it by talking about it. They fear that talking about the patient's impending death would hasten it by making it a reality. She cited the case of a couple, married for thirty years, who were not communicating with each other concerning the husband's terminal condition. The wife felt that she had to be "up" for her dying husband, but she did not feel "up"; she was frightened and anxious. The social work task in this case was to encourage the wife's expression of her feelings, and, at the same time to validate a sharing of those feelings with her husband so that he, in turn, could feel free to express any fears he might have to his wife. The social worker also observed that denial is a typical reaction to end-of-life situations and should not be challenged with certain patients or caregivers who might not be able to "get through the day" without a modicum of denial. In this regard, the appropriate social work approach is a function of a depth of understanding and empathy that can only be sustained by sharing with other hospice team members observations of her patients and their caregivers so that a concerted approach is assured. She expressed a sense of camaraderie with her hospice team members that enables her to reach out to hospice patients and their family networks so that no one is alone in the patient's end-of-life experience. Rather, everyone is on a journey together during which the social worker makes a difference by "being there and helping the patient and family understand what to expect" (Quigley, 2003). In this journey metaphor, the social worker is the tour guide who supports, reassures, informs, and facilitates the end-of-life process with sensitivity and skill.

## CAREGIVER STRESS

Stress is an accepted part of caring for older people. The primary caregiver must deal with stressors that those caring for patients who are recovering from acute illness may not face. The key difference is *recovery* of the patient. Older recipients of care, whether terminally ill or not, usually do not recover per se. They may reach a point where their health condition is managed so that they can avoid medical crises or acute episodes of chronic illness. However, the functionality of these care recipients typically is on a downward slope. The practice experience of this writer (S. R.) has been that the functional status of older people who are discharged from the hospital is usually more compromised than it was upon admission. Although medical science and technology are able to fix acute problems and manage chronicity for lengthy periods, elders' functional reserve is not necessarily protected or affected. Therefore, caregivers and elder care recipients need to be helped to deal with the primary stressor of that caregiving situation: the realization that limited improvement rather than complete recovery has to be the goal, and that convalescence may not include recovery of one's prior functional status. The role of social service is to ease this major stressor by helping caregivers to understand and accept not only what is beyond their capacity to affect but to understand the importance of emotional support.

Although the care recipients may not be able to recover their former level of functioning, it helps to know that with sensitive care, they can recover or sustain their emotional, feeling selves. The caregiving and social assistance task here is one of morale building. Of course, caregivers of Alzheimer's patients face what may seem to be insurmountable barriers in this regard. However, focusing caregiving objectives on emotional support can be effective.

### Case Study

*Practice experience reveals that emotional healing of Alzheimer's patients can happen when patients' recall past identities and accomplishments. At a social day program for Alzheimer's patients and their caregivers, a former professional singer vocalized beautifully; a former dermatologist (who recognized no one by name and increasingly could not remember faces of family caregivers) commented to a volunteer on her "beautiful skin." Further, he was able to discuss the basics of skin care with her and exhibited none of the agitation and palpable anxiety that was a part of his usual affect.*

## RESPITE CARE

It is hardly surprising that caregivers often develop burnout as well as physical and psychological problems that may compromise or even preclude their caregiving efforts. They themselves as a result will require help. This help may be in the form of respite care, or care for the caregiver (Tepper & Toner, 1993). Caregivers of terminally ill elderly or those with functional loss are better able to deal with major stressors if they are helped to seek respite opportunities in order to preserve their own physical and emotional well-being. Respite care—time away from the patient—is essential in a social care context that focuses almost solely on the needs of the care recipient. Support of the informal and professional caregiver(s) is often overlooked. Such support should be central to any social work with care recipients and their informal caregivers, with attention as well to the professional caregivers involved, including themselves! First, acknowledging caregivers' need for self-care should be given, followed by the identification and promotion of specific strategies for caregivers' attention to their own needs. With the application of medical technology to sustain life for longer and longer periods, research that examines the association between extended caregiving situations and caregiver well-being is abundant. Bookwala, Yee, and Schulz (2000) found that providing care to a person at the end of life was associated with the caregiver's decreased mental and physical health. Studies of caregivers found that higher levels of burden correlate with a worsening in quality of the caregiver–recipient relationship (Draper, Poulos, Poulos, & Erlich, 1995). Poor physical health was found to be more of a problem in women than in men as caregivers (Bookwala & Schultz, 2000). This reinforces the need for respite care and for the provision of supportive assistance for both caregiver and patient as a unit, and as discrete entities needing separate interventions. Chapters 2, 3, 5, 9, and 10 in this volume provide additional information on caregiver stress.

## GRIEF AND LOSS

Grief and loss are major end-of-life concerns for elders facing terminal illness and for their loved ones and caregivers. The sense of loss of a healthy past and all that is associated with that quality of life is common. This sense of loss typically may be expressed in overt mourning or depressed mood states, if not clinical depression.

Hospice social workers and others assigned to helping elderly end-of-life clients must first identify feelings and expressions of grief and loss and then apply their professional skills to help clients work through these emotions. In this connection, social work's principle of individualized assistance is essential. A person's experience of grief and loss is his or hers alone and though the stages of their grief experience may be generally predictable, the experience itself is an individual one. An important aspect of effective social work applicable to grief and loss is the worker's own attitudes and feelings about death and dying (Parry, 1989). In order to help clients in the process of accepting the absence of their loved one, social workers must first understand their own reactions to loss and mourning.

## BEREAVEMENT SUPPORT

The Medicare Hospice benefit includes twelve months of bereavement support services to surviving family and friends of patients. The hospice worker is typically responsible for the design and delivery of these services, which may be extended to bereaved persons in the community at large. Services to help survivors cope with their loss may include writing periodic letters of support (see Appendix 1 at the end of this book), sending educational material relating to coping with specific losses (parent, spouse), and providing ongoing informational or peer support groups that may operate from eight to ten weeks and are usually based on the prescreening and registration of participants. The American Association of Retired Persons offers a guide to the provision of support groups and a peer support telephone line, a website (www.aarp.org) with information about AARP grief and loss programs, and updated articles and resources relating to bereavement support needs.

Survivors whose bereavement experience interferes seriously with their ability to recover personal or familial equilibrium in the absence of their loved ones may be diagnosed with pathological grief response and may be referred for mental health interventions other than individual and group support counseling (which Medicare hospice benefits may or may not include in their bereavement support programs). This writer (S. R.) has developed an assessment form for the bereaved person's identification of behavioral or emotional indicators of pathological grief. See Appendix 2 at the end of this book.

## CONCLUSION

End-of-life issues are increasingly coming to the forefront of social service with the aging of the 65+ population. As the number of elderly with these concerns increases, so does the variety of life circumstances and personal characteristics of these elderly. Therefore, it is incumbent upon social workers and other professionals serving this population to develop relevant perspectives for their interventions that sufficiently take into account the multifaceted and individual expressions by older adults and their families of their end-of-life concerns. The authors hope that this chapter has contributed to such a perspective in the field of social service.

## REFERENCES

Ahronheim, J. G. (1997). End of life issues for very elderly women: Incurable and terminal illness. *Journal of the American Medical Woman's Association, 52*(3), 147–151.

Austin, B. J., & Fleisher, L. K. (2003). Financing end-of-life care: Challenges for an aging population. *Academy Health* (pp. 1–16). The Robert Wood Johnson HCFO Program.

Bookwala, J., & Schulz, E. (2000). A comparison of primary stressors, secondary stressors, and depressive symptoms between elderly caregiving husbands and wives: The caregiver health effects study. *Psychology and Aging, 15*(4), 607–616.

Bookwala, J., Yee, J., & Schulz, R. (2000). Caregiving and detrimental mental and physical health outcomes. In G. M. Williamson, P. A. Parmelee, & D. R. Shaffer (Eds.), *Physical illness and depression in older adults: A handbook of theory, research, and practice* (pp. 93–131). New York: Plenum.

Buntin, M. B., & Huskamp, H. (2002). What is known about the economics of end-of-life care for Medicare beneficiaries? *The Gerontologist, 42*, 40–48.

Burger, S. (2002). Palliative and end-of-life care: Patient and family concerns. *Caring for the Ages, 3*(7), 1–7.

Centers for Disease Control. (2003). Public health and aging: Trends in aging: The United States and worldwide. *Morbidity and Mortality Weekly Report, 52*(6), 101–106.

Draper, B. M., Poulos, R. G., Poulos, C. J., & Erlich, F. (1995). Risk factors for stress in elderly caregivers. *International Journal of Geriatric Psychiatry, 11*, 227–231.

Federal Forum on Aging Related Statistics. (2002). Current populations survey supplement. Available at www.agingstats.gov/tables

Gutheil, I., & Tepper, L. (1997). The aging family: Ethnic and cultural considerations. In E. P. Congress (Ed.), *Multicultural perspectives in working with families* (pp. 89–108). New York: Springer.

Hospice Association of America. (2003). Hospice: A historical perspective. *Hospice Association of America home page, 4*, 1–4.

Komaroff, A. L. (2002). *A guide to Alzheimer's disease* (pp. 36–37). (Special Health Report). Boston: Harvard Medical School Publications.

Levenson, S. (2002). Interdisciplinary approach: Dream team or nightmare. *Caring for the Ages, 3*(7).

Munley, A. (1983). A new context for death and dying. *The hospice alternative* (pp. 233–245). New York: Basic Books.

Parry, J. K. (1989). Transitions and reflections. *Social work theory and practice with the terminally ill* (pp. 105–121). New York: Haworth.

Quigley, M. (2003). Interview at Kershaw County Medical Center Hospice Program, Camden, SC.

Rea, N. K., Popeski, M., & Zinchiak, P. A. (2001). Older adult health report. *Health Status Indicator Project, Health Care Cost Summit,* PA: Erie County Department of Health. Available at http://www.ecdh.org

Smith, A., & Hetzel, L. (2001). *Census 2000 brief.* U.S. Department of Commerce: U.S. Census Bureau Economic and Statistics Administration (C2KBR/01-10).

Tepper, L. M., & Toner, J. A. (1993). *Respite care: Programs, problems and solutions.* Philadelphia: Charles.

U.S. Department of Health and Human Services. (2001). Healthy People 2010: Report of the Nation's Health Agenda. Washington, DC: U.S. Department of Health and Human Services.

# Part III

---

## Financial, Ethical, and Legal Issues in Elder Care

# 12

# Financing Health Care

## Thomas Campbell Jackson

M any of the interventions for older Americans described else-
where in this text carry a price tag, often a significant one
(Lubitz, Cai, Kramarow, & Lentzner, 2003). Partly by default
and partly in reflection of America's decentralized health care system,
funding for these costs is fragmented among diverse, overlapping—even
competing—financing mechanisms. Market and political forces contin-
uously interact to evoke adaptive behaviors by patients, providers, and
payers (a prime example being the transformation of Medicaid into
the primary payer of long-term care for the middle-class elderly).

The implications of haphazard financing are magnified for older
Americans, with their frequently fixed incomes. Frustrated by flaws in
their current coverage, they may still be apprehensive about changes
to it. Many will be confused by detailed insurance documents, and all
are understandably made anxious by conflicting media reports, adver-
tisements, and political grandstanding. But even as reform proposals
percolate through academia and government, individual elderly need
assistance *today*. Those who would serve them must know how to work
with existing programs and policies.

A single chapter could never untangle the Gordian knot of health
care finance, with all its economic, political, and historical dimensions.
Rather, this overview will highlight representative problems readers
will surely encounter (whether as providers of services or ultimately as
patients), and present an approach to thinking about insurance issues.
Resources listed at the chapter's end are a starting point for making
the detailed inquiries necessary to answer specific questions.

## THE REALITIES OF INSURANCE

The share of health-related costs paid for out of pocket by patients of
all ages has been falling for decades (Centers for Medicare & Medicaid

Services, 2003). Increasingly, the major source of funding is "insurance," a term often casually applied to a variety of arrangements for facilitating access to care.

Insurance is a means of transferring or pooling risk and/or its financial consequences. It is used in other spheres to deal with events that are rare and unpredictable, detrimental, generally beyond influence by the insured, and financially devastating—conditions not readily apparent in health care. For example, the need for care is often more of a certainty than a risk, particularly among the elderly. Most health services are desirable and actively sought out by patients or ordered by providers. *Moral hazard* is a term which describes how insurance changes the way we act. It refers to the interplay of behavior and immunity from certain consequences of that behavior, and like so much else, it is different where health care is concerned. Assured financing can be salutary when it increases access to needed services (McWilliams, Zaslavsky, Meara, & Ayanian, 2003), but it may also be wasteful or dangerous if it leads to inappropriate utilization. As an example, knowledge that our expenses are "covered" in the event of accident or illness may result in failure to take certain precautions conducive to good health. The uniqueness of health care is accentuated among the elderly, with their increased burden of morbidity, and helps account for many of the real and perceived shortcomings of current insurance arrangements.

Most working Americans obtain their health care through employment-based benefits. Though its origins predate World War II, this practice became common at that time as a way for employers to attract workers despite wage controls. Health costs paid by businesses are tax free to workers and tax deductible to employers, and both constituencies value this voluntary arrangement for leveraging compensation, despite lingering confusion over who precisely bears the cost. There is strong evidence, however, that employees pay for their benefits in the form of foregone wages (Pauly, 1997).

Still, this "tax preference" did little to address the health needs of people over age 65, and it remained for Medicare, the social insurance program for the elderly and disabled enacted in 1965, to assure them access to more than charity medical care. Related legislation like the Older Americans Act of the same year, which created the Administration on Aging and funded certain social, nutrition, and other initiatives, accelerated efforts to address the health care deficit among the elderly.

Over time, generous public and private funding fostered a cycle of ever more comprehensive benefits, rising prices, and increasing demand for broader coverage as protection from those costs. Even with massive entitlements and open-ended tax subsidies, health resources remain inescapably limited. Consequently, every health care paradigm entails rationing of funding, of care, or more typically both.

The federal Health Maintenance Organization (HMO) Act of 1973 created employer mandates for new service delivery models, and these eventually flourished as the private sector turned increasingly to managed care. Within Medicare itself, rapidly rising expenditures led to a change from cost-plus to prospective payment. Beginning in 1983, a system of Diagnosis Related Groups (DRGs) established new guidelines for reimbursement to hospitals. In 1991, a similar approach was adopted for reimbursing physicians.

Cost-benefit judgments, technology assessment, quality improvement, and other efforts to enhance equity and efficiency are increasingly important. Although they can be made more or less transparent to patient and provider (the first and second parties to a health care encounter), fundamental economic decision making cannot be eliminated, only shifted. Indeed, responsibility for these decisions is routinely—if often inadvertently—delegated to public or private plans sponsors. These third party payers weigh competing interests of employees, retirees, and dependents; unions, management and shareholders; taxpayers and politicians. They allocate resources, with some favoring "first dollar" coverage of efficacious and inexpensive preventive care, checkups, screenings, and so forth, and others a "last dollar" approach, leaving people responsible for more of the manageable smaller costs but shielding them from catastrophic expenses. Many elderly, especially the sick and vulnerable, are glad to have someone else make these decisions. Others—again, especially when sick—are loath to cede control. One person's freedom of choice is another's difficult decision.

In practice, sponsors themselves rely heavily on fiscal agents to stretch available funding, keep the cost of coverage down, minimize waste and abuse, and encourage desired behavior. Cost sharing (deductibles, copayments, and coinsurance). benefit limitations (categorical exclusions, restrictions on choice of providers, service limits, age guidelines, pre-existing condition exclusions, dollar caps on benefits), and eligibility restrictions are among the most common approaches. These measures are infinitely fungible, and just as caregivers have trouble keeping up with changing rules, so they should not assume that the insured has kept fully abreast of them either. Providers should take time to ask about coverage for contemplated services, and encourage patients to check with their insurer in advance so as to avoid unpleasant surprises.

## ISSUES FOR AGING WORKERS

Because health benefits are so closely tied to employment and age, transitions are virtually unavoidable. Switching jobs or moving to a new home often means a change in coverage, and many employees remain at an otherwise unsatisfactory job solely for the benefits. People should be very cautious when changing health plans, consulting plan representatives and thoroughly researching benefits (and current and likely future prices) wherever possible. This caution is especially applicable to the elderly. Health problems once evident may impact eligibility, and it may not be possible to regain certain coverage once it has been dropped.

Those who retire "early" (i.e., before Medicare eligibility) are often in a difficult situation; even if they have qualified for Medicare supplementary coverage from an employer, they may face a coverage gap until they reach age 65. COBRA, the federal Consolidated Omnibus Reconciliation Act of 1985, allows most employees and their dependents who would otherwise lose coverage under an employer's group plan to continue benefits for a period of time at their own expense. This can be costly, but group coverage may be cheaper or more comprehensive than non-group alternatives. COBRA can help those between jobs or early retirees awaiting Medicare eligibility for up to 18 months, and dependents who lose benefits when the policyholder enrolls in Medicare can buy this coverage for three years. Individuals already on Medicare when their right to COBRA arises may also continue group benefits (though Medicare is primary), and some do to retain drug or other benefits. COBRA regulations specify a strict timetable for steps to be taken by both employer and employee, and individuals are well advised to follow all rules and document their compliance. At the expiration of COBRA coverage it is often possible to "convert" from group to individual coverage through the same insurance plan, though prices and terms may be far less favorable.

It is increasingly common for people to work past age 65, whether by choice or necessity. The Age Discrimination in Employment Act of 1967 assured that the working aged would continue to enjoy the same health benefits offered to co-workers under age 65; if an employer offers health benefits to 20 or more employees, it must make them available to all employees regardless of age. Most people elect to continue this coverage if available, especially if the employer contributes toward the cost. Some also choose to begin paying Part B premiums, and use Medicare as secondary insurance. If so, coverage is limited by what Medicare would have paid and what the employer's plan approved. Moreover, signing up for Medicare Part B will trigger a six-month open enrollment period for purchasing Medicare Supplemental coverage. Alternatively, enrollment in Part B can be postponed until work ceases; no late enrollment penalties apply, and the opportunity to sign up for Medicare Supplement policies without underwriting is merely postponed. A few older workers elect Medicare as their primary insurer, though their employer is not permitted to contribute in any way to the cost of supplemental coverage.

In spite of Americans' increasing "health span," age 65 remains an insurance watershed, and there is no requirement that employers continue benefits for retired workers. Many do, often as part of collective bargaining agreements, but rising costs have convinced some plans to scale back such coverage (Fronstin & Salisbury, 2003). This trend accelerated after a 1993 accounting regulation required employers to reflect the cost of retiree medical benefits in reporting corporate earnings, a change that drastically increased the attention paid to the cost of such benefits.

## MEDICARE

Americans frustrated with the limits and cost of coverage during their working years often look forward to retirement, when "I'll be on Medicare and everything will be simple." Despite perennial budget and service challenges, the federal health insurance program for those age 65 and over (and adults with certain disabilities) remains exceedingly popular with beneficiaries and most providers, covering some 41 million beneficiaries with total expenditures of $266 billion in 2002.

Medicare is basically divided into two parts, each with its own funding sources, cost sharing arrangements, rules, and politics. "Hospital Insurance" (Part A) covers most inpatient services and is funded by mandatory payroll tax deductions (2.9% of wages, half paid by the employee and half by the employer), as well as cost sharing by beneficiaries. Those who receive monthly Social Security benefits, as well as their spouses and some former spouses, are automatically eligible for Medicare upon turning 65. (Others who don't have the work contribution history to qualify automatically for coverage may purchase the coverage, which is another source of funding.)

"Medical Insurance" (Part B) is voluntary, and covers doctors' fees, outpatient hospital services, and other costs. Funding comes 75% from general government revenues and 25% from enrollees' monthly premiums (currently $66.60, which most beneficiaries have deducted from their Social Security checks). Higher income beneficiaries will be charged a larger Part B premium beginning in 2007. Those who do not enroll in Part B when they are first eligible may do so during the first calendar quarter of each year for coverage beginning the following July. Unless the delay in enrollment is due to continued employment, however, there will be a permanently higher monthly premium attached to the coverage.

"Medicare Advantage" (formerly Medicare + Choice or "Part C") offers alternative plan designs for receiving benefits generally similar to those in Parts A and B, and occasionally more comprehensive. Prescription drug coverage recently enacted may be called Part D.

## OVERVIEW OF CURRENT MEDICARE BENEFITS

### Part A

1.   *Hospital (Inpatient) Care:* Medicare's coverage for acute hospital stays is comprehensive, and includes room and board, drugs, nursing care, equipment, lab tests and x-rays, as well as ICU, OR, and other specialty unit charges. The first 60 days of a stay (most are much shorter) are covered in full after a deductible of $876. (Hospital coverage is reckoned in "benefit periods," which start with admission and run to 60 days after discharge. A separate deductible is payable for each benefit period, but not required for readmissions within 60 days.) Coverage from the 61st to the 90th day requires a daily copayment of $219, and for those rare longer confinements, 60 "lifetime reserve" days are available subject to a daily copayment of $438. Stays longer than 150 days are not covered at all by Medicare. Inpatient psychiatric care is covered in full after the deductible, but limited to 190 days in a lifetime. The cost of blood is covered after the first three pints.

2.   *Skilled Nursing Facility (SNF) Care:* Medicare covers up to 100 days of SNF benefits in each benefit period, but only following a hospital stay of at least three days for the underlying condition, and only if SNF care commences within 30 days of discharge. The first twenty days are covered in full, but copayments of $109.50 are required for the 21st through the 100th day. All coverage requires a doctor's orders, and custodial care is essentially excluded.

3.   *Post-Acute Home Health Care:* When ordered by a doctor and provided by a Medicare-approved agency, coverage is available to homebound patients requiring intermittent skilled nursing care or physical, occupational, or speech therapy. The coverage can extend to health aides, durable medical equipment, and some very limited assistance with ADLs.

4.   *Hospice Care:* For those reaching the end stages of a terminal illness, Medicare covers broad palliative care, with little or no cost

sharing. Care is typically rendered in the home, but may include brief hospital stays to stabilize or give respite to caregivers.

## Part B

1.  *Physicians' and surgeons' services:* The costs of care at the hospital, doctor's office, or home are covered, as are anesthesia, radiology, and pathology, as well as second opinions and other services.

2.  *Outpatient hospital care:* The coverage for outpatient hospital care includes the emergency room, clinics, and blood transfusions.

3.  *Physical and Occupational Therapy:* Rehabilitation costs provided by physical therapists and occupational therapists are covered when ordered by a doctor.

4.  *Home Care:* Certain types of home care that are not connected to a stay in a hospital or SNF is covered in full.

5.  *Psychiatric care:* Mental health services are covered 80% in a hospital outpatient setting, and 50% in a doctor's office.

6.  *Other coverage:* Coverage under Part B includes Durable Medical Equipment, ambulance trips, x-rays, and blood (at 80% of the approved amount), certain laboratory tests, mammograms, pap smears, and influenza and pneumonia vaccines (covered in full), and a variety of other items and services.

## Prescription Drug Coverage Legislation

As this volume went to press, a number of changes to Medicare had just been signed into law under the Medicare Prescription Drug, Improvement, and Modernization Act of 2003, most notably coverage for prescription drugs. A voluntary outpatient prescription drug benefit will be offered by competing private companies beginning in 2006 (with preliminary benefits phased in beginning in 2004). Coverage will be subject to a somewhat elaborate arrangement of deductibles and co-insurance, with provisions for catastrophic coverage and extra subsidies directed at those with lower incomes.Chronic disease management initiatives are added, along with new screening tests and a single checkup at enrollment. Part C is reorganized to promote Preferred Provider Organizations, though direct competition between Traditional Medicare and private alternatives does not begin for a number of years. The Act provides $88 billion in subsidies to dissuade employers from reducing coverage under existing Medicare programs. Nothing in the act appears likely to alter the fundamental challenges facing the program, however.

## MEDICARE'S GUARDED PROGNOSIS

Sadly, Medicare itself does not exhibit the robustness that increasingly characterizes its 34.6 million beneficiaries over age 65. Driven by demographics and increased intensity of utilization, program expenditures as a percentage of the Gross Domestic Product are expected to at least double from 2.6% in 2002 to 5.3% by 2035. Although projections differ, the Hospitalization Insurance trust fund will likely begin to decline within a decade or so, and could be depleted by 2026 (Boards of Trustees, 2003). Although access to general revenues means funding is not as directly constrained for Part B, there, too, expenditures are expected to outstrip economic growth with ominous implications for enrollee premiums. Medicare's popularity with physicians waxes and wanes with reimbursement rates, and these are periodically adjusted to reflect budget constraints on the one hand, and declining provider participation on the other. More broadly, it remains to be seen whether the baby boomers, famed for taking control of their lives in general and their health in particular, will be as satisfied with the program as were their parents, in light of the increased cost sharing and benefit restrictions that loom.

## EXISTING GAPS IN "UNIVERSAL" COVERAGE

With its wide enrollment and extensive provider participation, Medicare could be described as a "targeted universal health care program," but despite comprehensive benefits, even Medicare falls short of total protection. Indeed, the program was never intended to cover all of the medical costs of the elderly, and today covers only about half of the typical beneficiary's expenses (Fronstin & Salisbury, 2003), a lower fraction than when it was enacted. Out-of-pocket health spending averages about 19% of income for all Medicare beneficiaries, though the figure can be much higher for those who are poorer, older, or sicker, and lower for those in a managed care plan (American Association of Retired Persons, 1997). Long-term care, most preventive care, regular dental and foot care, hearing aids or eyeglasses, and services outside of the United States are not covered. Medicare generally does not pay, or pays on a secondary basis only, for services covered by other private policies or government programs. Coverage for many of the services listed above is limited, and cost sharing through premiums, deductibles, coinsurance, and excess doctors' charges is potentially unlimited.

Although 13.5% of beneficiaries have traditional Medicare alone, the majority carry additional coverage. Fully 32.4% have additional coverage by virtue of an employer's benefit plan (Goldman & Zissimopoulos, 2003). Those with particularly low incomes—7.7% of Medicare enrollees (Goldman & Zissimopoulos)—qualify for special assistance under Medicaid, the joint federal/state health program for the poor. For "Qualified Medicare Beneficiaries" (those at or below the federal poverty line) Medicaid can pay Medicare's premiums, coinsurance, and deductibles. An individual with income above the federal poverty level (but no more than 20% above) can still have the monthly Part B premium paid by his or her state as a Specified Low-Income Beneficiary. Other programs of assistance, including some services not covered by Medicare at all, may be available under Medicaid, depending on the state.

Some 15% of elderly Medicare beneficiaries have additional coverage by virtue of enrollment in a managed care plan (Goldman & Zissimopoulos, 2003), though this assumes a willingness to sacrifice some choice of providers and to risk untimely closure of the plan. Provisions in the Medicare Prescription Drug, Improvement, and Modernization Act are intended to strengthen Medicare managed care arrangements to avoid the plan closures that have been common (Lake & Brown, 2002).

Approximately 32% of enrollees purchase a Medicare supplemental or "Medigap" policy (Goldman & Zissimopoulos, 2003). In most states there are ten approved plans, with benefits standardized to facilitate comparison. Prices vary by location, benefit package (not all are available in all areas), and policy design. All Medigap plans cover a basic group of benefits, including the hospital coinsurance and an additional year of hospital coverage beyond Medicare's limit, as well as the Part B coinsurance. Some offer additional coverage, most commonly excess charges under Part B, and prescription drugs (although this coverage is rather costly and limited). Medicare beneficiaries can sign up to buy any of these plans, regardless of health, during a six-month window beginning when they sign up for Medicare Part B; enrollment at other times may be subject to underwriting or other restrictions. Under the Medicare Prescription Drug, Improvement, and Modernization Act, new supplement policies will be added in 2006, though no new policies with drug coverage will be sold at that point.

"Medicare Select" policies are similar to Medigap policies, and offer less expensive coverage in exchange for use of providers participating in a network.

The Veterans Administration runs the largest health care system in the nation, and a third of the population—veterans, and sometimes their dependents or survivors—are entitled to a variety of benefits through it. Though beneficiaries are increasingly prioritized for financial reasons, those with service-related conditions or particular financial need may be able to access significant assistance through the VA. In addition, as of 2001 a program called "TRICARE for Life" extends Medicare supplemental benefits to military retirees and eligible dependents. The coverage is free and includes prescription drugs.

## LONG-TERM CARE FINANCING

Of all the challenges in financing health care for an aging America, one of the more daunting is long-term care (LTC). Overall growth of the elderly population (including the particularly rapid increase in the number of the oldest Americans), the rise in chronic disease in all age categories, and budgetary constraints at the federal and state levels are aligning to bring about a "perfect storm" crisis in funding this type of care.

Long-term care encompasses services ranging from intensive nursing and other skilled care to personal and purely custodial care. It is rendered in a variety of settings, such as patients' own homes, Assisted Living Facilities (ALFs), and Skilled Nursing Facilities (SNFs/ Nursing Homes). Triggers for LTC include needing assistance with activities of daily living (ADLs) and cognitive impairment. Though much of the need for these types of services is accounted for by those under 65 as the result of injury or chronic illness and some will be needed by older patients on a limited basis (as for rehabilitation after an acute condition), the bulk of the need is represented by patients whose care needs routinely extend months, years, or indefinitely, especially in nursing homes. It is commonly estimated that half of those over age 65 today will eventually need LTC of one kind or another, and the vast majority of the oldest will require some sort of assistance on an ongoing basis.

Widespread ignorance prevails regarding the fact that these services are not covered by health insurance, Medicare, or Medigap. (As previously described, Medicare's coverage is limited to post-acute stays of 100 days or less.) In practice, most LTC is uncompensated, provided informally by family or friends, but the greatest pecuniary costs are associated with nursing homes. Medicaid covers some 70% of SNF residents, paying almost 80% of all patient days. The program's size and limited funds are reflected in reimbursement rates often below a facility's operating costs. By law, any Medicaid contribution to the cost of a patient day means the facility can collect no more than Medicaid's own meager rate in total, and this pressure is a major cause of nursing home bankruptcies. In fact, many SNFs are only able to remain open as a result of Medicare rehabilitation stays and high charges to private payers. (Patients who can spend their own money, at least for a while, sometimes find that they are able to gain access to more desirable facilities. About half of those who go to nursing homes begin paying something out of pocket, but most eventually go on to Medicaid.)

This arrangement is a big problem for Medicaid, for providers of care, and for those looking to that program for coverage. Medicaid was established alongside Medicare in 1965 to provide health services to the poor. It is a state administered program, funded jointly by the federal and state (and in some instances local) governments. Although specific numbers vary by state, Medicaid applies both asset and income tests to prospective beneficiaries. In short, with certain notable exceptions such as a home, you must be poor, or make yourself essentially poor, to qualify.

This is inherently undesirable to most people. One result is extensive demand for and practice of "Medicaid planning" to divest or shield assets in preparation for qualifying for public assistance. This practice may suit older Americans whose sole goal is to leave an estate (and doubtless pleases some greedy children as well), but has severe consequences. Because Medicaid pays for little LTC outside of nursing homes, this artificial depletion of assets essentially restricts the older patient needing care to that setting. Serving as the primary payer for LTC has stressed Medicaid enormously. Overall Medicaid expenditures are expected to exceed those of Medicare for the first time in 2004. As the largest item in many state budgets, Medicaid effectively crowds out other worthy government programs, and has an increasingly difficult time achieving its primary mission of assuring the poor access to health care.

Just as the World War II generation was behind the expansion of employment-based benefits, Medicare and Medicaid, so the baby boomers are driving the evolution of LTC. We are still in the early stages of this development, and a couple of decades remain until most boomers reach ages needing assistance. Already, however, the growth of alternative care settings, the increasing demand for personal control, and rising expectations reflect the impact of this cohort. As a likely indication of future trends, the percentage of the oldest old in nursing homes is already declining as other options arise, albeit on a private-pay basis. The institutionalized population is frailer and poorer.

Many long-term SNF residents require essentially custodial services, and could be cared for at home with proper support. Unfortunately, few states can afford to expand Medicaid coverage to include care outside nursing homes, with the result that Medicaid's "institutional bias" constrains those who may not need or want to, to live in an SNF. Increased private funding is necessary to help the elderly pay for insurance or care itself. Options include reverse mortgages to tap accumulated home equity (over a trillion dollars by some estimates), life insurance policies incorporating LTC benefits, settlements on life insurance policies, and annuities. The most promising vehicle may be private insurance for LTC.

## LONG-TERM CARE INSURANCE

The public's faulty assumptions about Medicare coverage for LTC, and the existence of Medicaid as payer of last resort, have hindered development of insurance for LTC. Additionally, Americans tend to think of health-related expenses in terms of employment benefits, and because this type of coverage was until recently not offered through the workplace, it was simply not on the radar of working people who are typically in the best position financially, and from a health perspective, to purchase affordable coverage.

Early LTC insurance policies were typically quite restrictive, usually requiring prior hospitalization or covering services in institutional settings only, and they often were a poor value. Today, the market is developing rapidly as the result of growing numbers and sophistication of buyers, increased industry experience, greater competition, and tax incentives.

One example of the latter is the Health Insurance Portability and Accountability Act (HIPAA). Beginning in 1997, the HIPAA established criteria for federally qualified LTC policies, including what benefits must be paid, what triggers coverage, and what options have to be made available to buyers. Premiums for qualified policies are deductible within certain limits, and benefits are tax free. Some insurers offer "Nonqualified" policies, which lack tax benefits but are sometimes easier to obtain and may in some instances be more suitable to a particular person's needs.

In addition, half of the states encourage the purchase of LTC insurance with tax deductions or credits. Five have also established "Partnership Plans" whereby the purchase of a qualifying insurance policy protects an equivalent dollar amount of assets that would otherwise need to be spent down prior to Medicaid eligibility.

Long-term care may be sold on an individual or group basis, and is increasingly included among employment-based benefit offerings. In 2000, the federal government as an employer made LTC insurance available as an optional benefit for certain current and former federal workers—perhaps 20 million potential customers.

As with health insurance, LTC insurers rely on a variety of utilization and cost controls. Policies vary in what will trigger benefits and what types of services are covered (though a doctor's orders are a common requirement). Benefit limits may be expressed in dollars, duration and level of care, and locations approved for covered services. Waiting or "elimination" periods are akin to a deductible, and may apply after a triggering event but before benefits are payable. As with any other major financial commitment, careful research is in order.

The benefits of LTC insurance are manifold, however, and include empowerment of the elderly, much needed cash infusions into SNFs (and the quality improvements this makes possible), strengthening the Medicaid program and easing the burden on state budgets, and enabling families to purchase adult day care, respite care, and professional assistance as necessary.

Buying LTC if you can afford it is a very good idea, and the earlier the better is a good rule of thumb. Delaying the purchase of insurance is not likely to bring savings as higher premiums will apply. Moreover, those who wait run the risk of not qualifying for coverage at all should health problems arise.

The goal of most Americans is to be able to age in place, or at least in a place of their choice. This happy arrangement is dependent on several things: an appropriate senior-friendly environment, a healthy spouse or other friend or relative, available transportation, and other resources. In the absence of these, personal resources—whether in the form of insurance, savings, or reverse mortgages—can provide the option of paying for services in the most appropriate or desirable settings.

The prevailing welfare model for funding LTC is highly dysfunctional. It is both demeaning and conducive to elder abuse. By requiring divestiture of most assets as the price of Medicaid coverage it disenfranchises the elderly and effectively denies them the comfort and dignity that come with some control over one's situation.

## CONCLUSION

After spending years learning the complexities of their chosen specialty, caregivers often see the details of health insurance as a mere annoyance, but some familiarity with financial issues is necessary to be an effective advocate for aging patients and clients. Though not always easy, it will ultimately be more productive to deal with payers as the patient's designated (or de facto) agents—as partners in caring for patients—rather than as adversaries.

Whereas old age was once only a hope or sometimes a fear, today it is more of an expectation, albeit one only gradually reflected in public policy and market responses. Though the particulars of financing health care for the growing older population will continue to evolve, the basic economics and need for tradeoffs will not.

The need for care in old age is no risk, but a certainty we must prepare for, as individuals and as a society. Public resources are likely to be increasingly strained, and it seems safe to say that many future medical advances will be available only to those in a position to pay for them privately. We can empower the elderly by helping them prepare for the financial implications of old age during their working years, making sure they retain control of resources saved over a lifetime, and assisting them in accessing the manifold benefits public policy confers.

## REFERENCES

American Association of Retired Persons (AARP). (1997). *Out of pocket health spending by Medicare beneficiaries age 65 and older: 1997 projections.* # 9705. Washington, DC: Author. Available at http://research.aarp.org/health/9705_pocket.pdf

Boards of Trustees of the Federal Hospital Insurance and Federal Supplementary Medical Insurance Trust Funds. (2003). *Annual report, 2003.* Baltimore: Centers for Medicare & Medicaid Services.

Centers for Medicare & Medicaid Services (MS), Office of the Actuary, National Health Statistics Group. (2003). Table 4. Available at http://cms.hhs.gov/statistics/nhe/historical/t4.asp

Fronstin, P., & Salisbury, D. (2003). *Retiree health benefits: Savings needed to fund health care in retirement.* Washington, DC: Employee Benefit Research Institute.

Goldman, D. P., & Zissimopoulos, J. M. (2003). High out-of-pocket health care spending by the elderly. *Health Affairs, 22,* 194–202.

Lake, T., & Brown, R. (2002). *Medicare + choice withdrawals: Understanding key factors.* Menlo Park, CA: Henry J. Kaiser Family Foundation/Mathmatica Policy Research, Inc.

Lubitz, J., Cai, L., Kramarow, E., & Lentzner, H. (2003). Health, life expectancy, and health care spending among the elderly. *New England Journal of Medicine, 349,* 1048–1055.

McWilliams, J. M., Zaslavsky, A. M., Meara, E., & Ayanian, J. Z. (2003). Impact of Medicare coverage on basic clinical services for previously uninsured adults. *Journal of the American Medical Association, 290*(6), 757–764.

Pauly, M. A. (1997). *Health benefits at work: An economic and political analysis of employment based health insurance.* Ann Arbor, MI: University of Michigan Press.

# 13

# Issues in Elder Law

## Marshall B. Kapp

### Case Study

*Mrs. Jones is an 85-year-old widow from New York in previously good health who has suffered a massive stroke while visiting her daughter in California and has been rushed to St. Vincent's Hospital. Despite being subjected to aggressive medical efforts, Mrs. Jones is a patient in the hospital intensive care unit three days later in what her physicians (none of whom she had ever met before) describe as a permanent vegetative state with no realistic hope of recovering any cognition. She is flanked by her California daughter, who wants to follow the physicians' recommendation and discontinue all life-prolonging medical interventions, and a son to whom Mrs. Jones has not spoken in ten years who has flown in from Texas to demand that "everything" be done to keep his mother alive indefinitely. Prior to her stroke, Mrs. Jones had neither executed any type of formal advance medical directive nor spoken to anyone about her future treatment preferences. The physicians need someone who can make some definitive decisions about her treatment at this time and, anxious about their own liability risks, tell Mrs. Jones's adult children that they will either need to resolve their disagreement amicably or initiate a court action to obtain a legal ruling to guide the course of action.*

The "law" is the body of enforceable rules and prohibitions that is established by a jurisdiction's constitution, legislature, administrative agencies, and courts, as well as the processes that have been put in place to interpret and apply those rules. The law embodies and reflects important social attitudes, and orders and implements actions by society, thereby exerting a major influence on the lives of older persons in a variety of ways. The scenario described above represents one type of situation in which the legal system, in terms of its substantive principles and its decision-making processes, affects older persons and those who care about and for them. As the population increasingly ages, such circumstances inevitably will multiply.

## BACKGROUND

The burgeoning of elder law as a separate specialty area of legal study and practice is a relatively recent phenomenon (Frolik, 2002). Legal services for older persons are available from an array of private attorneys (on either a paid or pro bono basis) and public interest attorneys (Thomas & Ingham, 2003). Graduate and undergraduate programs offer focused courses and other educational experiences in this sphere (Kapp, 2001), specialized textbooks (Frolik & Barnes, 2003; Dayton, Gallanis, & Wood, 2003), practice handbooks (Frolik & Kaplan, 2003), and specialty journals and books in the popular press (American Bar Association, 1998). National and state organizations such as the National Academy of Elder Law Attorneys have proliferated and prospered.

The content of elder law is broad and (as is true for most of the topics covered in this book) highly interdisciplinary. Topics falling within this category entail, but are not limited to, the legal facets of Social Security retirement and disability benefits; other federal and state benefit programs; private pensions and other retirement issues; Medicare and Medicaid, including asset sheltering and divestiture for eligibility purposes, as well as private insurance coverage (see chapter 12); housing arrangements (see chapters 3 and 4), including landlord concerns and property tax assessments and exemptions; financial management (such as trusts) and estate planning; medical treatment decision making and advance medical planning; mental incapacity and judicial and non-judicial forms of substitute decision making; elder abuse, neglect, and exploitation (see chapter 15); employment discrimination; tax counseling; and rights as service and product consumers. Brief discussion of a few of these topics is presented below.

## MEDICAL DECISION MAKING AND ADVANCE PLANNING

As illustrated by the case of Mrs. Jones, medical decision making is one arena in which the legal parameters may substantially affect the quality, and indeed the very existence, of an older person's life. If Mrs. Jones could presently speak for herself competently, the law (through the informed consent doctrine) would assure her of the right to make her own choices concerning medical care. However, she is not currently capable of exercising that right autonomously.

To maximize the likelihood of continued control over their own medical treatment, older persons should anticipate future situations in which crucial medical decisions must be made, but when the individual may not be capable at that moment of making and communicating treatment preferences reached through a rational decision-making process. The two most important legal instruments available for advance health care planning are living wills and durable powers of attorney (Mishkin, Mezey, & Ramsey, 1995). Every state has enacted legislation that authorizes decisionally capable adults to execute either or both of these formal advance planning instruments.

## The Living Will

A living will is a kind of instruction directive in which adults who currently have decisional capacity document in writing their future desires regarding medical treatment. Forms for one's particular jurisdiction may be obtained from state medical and legal associations. It is not feasible to anticipate every conceivable future medical contingency; therefore, many individuals prefer to execute an alternative type of document in which the person identifies chosen values (for example, as the desire to live as long as possible without any consideration of costs to the family), rather than listing specific medical interventions to be provided or avoided. This type of directive often is referred to as a "Values History," and the widely disseminated Five Wishes form is one example of this approach to advance planning.

## The Durable Power of Attorney

A durable power of attorney (DPOA) for health care, on the other hand, is a written document created by a competent adult that nominates another person to act as a proxy or agent, ordinarily termed an "attorney-in-fact," with authority to make particular decisions on behalf of the patient if the patient becomes mentally incapacitated. The DPOA as an advance planning proxy instrument is most useful for people who have someone whom they can trust, and who is likely to be available to fulfill this function. Filling out a written form for this purpose, though, should be supplemented by timely, open communication with the designated agent, so that decisions made in the future are congruent with the patient's actual values and preferences. In the absence of effective communication, a person cannot automatically assume that the proxy will guess correctly what the patient would want to occur in specific future medical circumstances.

## Other Types of Advances Directives

Advance directives in the U.S. were given a major boost by Congressional enactment in 1990 of the federal Patient Self-Determination Act (PSDA). This legislation (42 United States code § 1395cc [a]) imposes on institutional and organization health care providers participating in the Medicare and Medicaid programs the following requirements (among others):

1.  The provider must develop and give to new patients or their surrogates a written policy explaining how that provider handles advance directives. This policy must be consistent with applicable state law but otherwise may reflect particular organizational values.
2.  The provider must ask, at or before the time of admission or enrollment, whether the patient has a currently valid advance directive.
3.  If there is no currently valid advance directive and the patient still is decisionally capable, the provider must ask whether that patient would like to execute an advance directive at that time.

Another type of advance directive for medical purposes is the "Do Not" order. "Do Not" orders written by an attending physician to other participants on the health care team are prospectively made decisions to withdraw or withhold certain kinds of medical interventions from a particular patient. Orders with potential significance for older patients, especially those living and/or receiving services in long-term care environments, are Do Not Resuscitate (DNR) (instructions by the physician not to initiate attempts at cardiopulmonary resuscitation (CPR) in the contingency of cardiac arrest), Do Not Hospitalize, and Do Not Treat.

From a legal perspective, Do Not orders should be governed by the same substantive and procedural rules that apply to other kinds of medical treatment decisions. Gerontological professionals should encourage older persons to initiate discussion with their physicians and families about the issues raised by Do Not orders and other possible treatment controversies in a timely, honest fashion. The older health care consumer has a right to expect adequate, current information about foreseeable benefits and burdens. A Do Not choice may be revoked or altered at any time, in light of changes in a patient's physical or mental condition that might modify the likely benefit/burden ratio presented by different treatment options.

When a patient is not presently capable of making decisions but has neglected to execute a valid advance medical directive earlier, decision-making power may devolve from the patient to another person by operation of a statute, regulation, or judicial precedent. In the majority of states, family consent statutes codify legal authority empowering specifically designated relatives to make certain kinds of medical choices for incapacitated individuals who have not executed an advance directive. Older individuals who fail to execute timely advance directives should be encouraged to learn about the usual legal progression of decision-making authority in their respective states, to make certain that the normal process is consistent with their own wishes and to take action if it is not.

Even in the absence of family consent statutes, courts in many states have formally recognized the power of a family member to exert an incapacitated person's decision-making prerogatives on that person's behalf. Many of these judicial decisions explicitly establish legal precedent for families to take on the proxy role in future cases without any requirement to obtain prior court authorization. Traditionally, even when there is neither an advance directive nor any specific controlling statute, regulation, or court order delegating authority to a decisionally incapacitated person's proxy decision maker, families have been accepted and relied on as surrogate decision makers as a matter of widely known and implicitly accepted medical custom.

Sometimes, however, something more than informal substitute decision making by the family and health care team may be necessary to respond to a problematic situation. Relatives may disagree with each other about the optimal course of medical treatment for their family member. They may make choices that appear to serve the earlier expressed or implied wishes of the patient poorly or that clearly seem to be contrary to the patient's best interests. The family may demand a course of behavior that seriously interferes with the physician's or facility's sense of moral responsibility. When such situations occur, the involved parties may need to petition a court to appoint a guardian or conservator with the authority to make decisions for the incapacitated patient.

Older persons ought to be urged to minimize the possibility of this sort of disharmonious scenario by engaging in timely, thoughtful family discussions and advance medical planning and documentation. Such planning, designed to maximize individual control in the future, is especially advisable for older persons who no longer have meaningful relationships with any relatives or others, and who hence might otherwise end up in jeopardy when questions of legal authority arise.

## FINANCIAL DECISION MAKING AND PLANNING

Financial or estate planning is an area with significant ramifications for an older person's quality of life, the range of residential (Kapp, 2002) and medical choices available to that person, and the person's ability to bestow a financial legacy on others while still alive and after death. Among other things, a person's failure to initiate financial planning at an opportune time may imperil that individual's later eligibility for certain public benefits such as Medicaid coverage for long-term care. Moreover, all financial planning decisions, whether made consciously or by default, carry important tax implications that may impact the future financial well-being of individuals and their heirs.

Comprehensive estate planning has a number of facets, with particulars depending on an individual's assets, family circumstances, and preferences. An ideal estate planning team would consist of an expert attorney, accountant, investment advisor, and insurance agent, all of whom would work in concert to promote the client's best interests.

In most cases, the centerpiece of an estate plan is a testamentary will. A will is a legal document, executed by a decision-capable adult (the testator), that directs the distribution of that adult's personal and real property after death. It also specifies an executor (or administrator or personal representative, with terminology varying somewhat among jurisdictions) to carry out the testator's wishes regarding the distribution. All people with any assets who care about their eventual distribution should consider signing a testamentary will. When a person dies, the terms of the will are implemented under judicial supervision through the process of probate.

Various forms of trust arrangements are available to help accomplish specific financial objectives held by a person. There are two basic kinds of trusts: revocable and irrevocable. Revocable trusts may be changed at any time, and usually the person who sets up the trust (the "trustor" or "settlor") can act as both a trustee and a beneficiary. By contrast, irrevocable trusts cannot be revoked or changed once they are established.

Within these two fundamental categories, there exist myriad variations. Trusts are categorized according to when they are created, who owns and benefits from the assets and income, how assets and income are distributed, and sundry other factors. Depending on circumstances, among the particular types of trust that an older person might consider are the following: credit-shelter trust, disclaimer trust, marital deduction trust, living or inter vivos trust, life insurance trust, qualified personal residence trust, charitable remainder trust, charitable lead trust, and generation-skipping trust.

A different type of financial planning strategy is the concept of joint property ownership. An older person could add the name of a spouse, adult child, or anyone else to a checking, savings, or other financial asset account. Such a move may facilitate banking transactions. Joint ownership arrangements involving two or more names on a single account include joint tenancy with right of survivorship and tenancy in common. However, only joint tenancy with right of survivorship allows one joint tenant to automatically receive the assets left in the account when the other person dies, without having to struggle through the expensive and time-consuming probate process and pay the otherwise associated estate taxes.

Some joint accounts allow either property owner to transact business and execute financial instruments; others require the agreement and signatures of all joint owners for any transactions; still others prohibit any single owner from unilaterally withdrawing funds. Local laws and banking practices set limits on what arrangements are permissible. In any situation, entering into a joint ownership status is predicated on a high level of trust in the judgment and honesty of those with whom one is sharing ownership.

Another type of financial planning available to many older persons is giving assets away, while one still can, to family members, friends, or nonprofit charitable organizations. Giving such financial gifts, though, may raise important implications regarding tax liability and eligibility for Medicaid and other means-tested government benefit programs.

In most jurisdictions, the law gives individuals the right to financially preplan their own funerals. Paying in advance for one's funeral gives one the opportunity to control significant details of that event and unburdens the family from needing to hassle with those arrangements, or substitutes for the absence of family and friends in making certain that one's last directions are respected. Before engaging in funeral preplanning, people should verify the right to cancel the agreement in the event that one moves or has a change of heart about these arrangements. Money paid in advance should be deposited only into a trust or escrow account managed by the funeral director.

Regulations of the Federal Trade Commission (FTC) require funeral directors to disclose to the client specific information about the funeral and to avoid involvement in unfair business practices. FTC rules are intended to protect the rights of individuals who preplan their own funerals, as well as those of relatives or friends of deceased persons who did not preplan. Most states have their own respective statutory counterparts to the FTC regulations, and state and federal laws apply concurrently.

## GUARDIANSHIP AND ITS ALTERNATIVES

The main legal and pragmatic devices for planning ahead, medically and financially, have been outlined above. When planning has not occurred and the concerned person becomes seriously cognitively impaired and therefore unable to make legally valid decisions, the locus of official decision-making authority must be clarified (for example, decisions about risky medical interventions or major financial transactions). In such circumstances, the mechanism most likely to be used to make decision-making power legally unambiguous is guardianship (Zimny & Grossberg, 1998). Guardianship is a legal relationship, established by a state court, between a ward (the person whom the court has found to be incompetent to make certain kinds of decisions) and a guardian (the individual or agency whom the court appoints as the substitute decision maker for the ward). Terminology regarding this relationship varies among the states; in California, for instance, the court-appointed surrogate is called a conservator.

The foundation of guardianship law is the doctrine of *parens patriae*, the inherent authority and responsibility of a compassionate society to act, even over objection if necessary, to protect people who are unable to fend for themselves. Hence, rather than simply abandoning seriously cognitively impaired persons in the name of an autonomy that does not truly exist for them, to make harmful decisions or neglect their fundamental needs, the state may exercise its power to safeguard even reluctant disabled individuals from the consequences of their own bad judgment.

When a court appoints a guardian to make surrogate decisions for a person who has been judged incompetent, the ward no longer has the authority to make those decisions that have been delegated to the guardian. Historically, society has imposed guardianship on an all-or-nothing basis; an alleged incapacitated person either was found globally capable, in which case that person retained all decision-making powers except those explicitly delegated to someone else, or globally incompetent, in which case the person was declared a ward and basically completely disenfranchised in terms of decision-making power. By contrast, the modern trend embodied in most states' guardianship statutes is toward legislative and judicial recognition of the concept of limited or partial, rather than plenary or total, guardianship. This concept is built around the decision-specific nature of mental capacity and the consequent ability of some people to make certain kinds of choices (for instance, whether or not to permit the taking of an x-ray) rationally but not others (such as whether to undergo major, risky surgery). Under a limited or partial guardianship order, a guardian is empowered to make only those kinds of decisions that the court determines the ward to be unable to make personally, but not other kinds of decisions. Modern judges are encouraged to distinguish as closely as possible between those domains where even a minimal level of capacity is lacking and those where, with sufficient assistance and support, the individual might be able to engage in a rational decision-making process. This more focused approach reflects the constitutional law principle, emanating from the Fourteenth Amendment Due Process clause, that, when an individual is not currently able to act autonomously, decisions should be made and acted on for the individual in the least intrusive, least restrictive manner reasonably available.

A major problem often occurs when a seriously cognitively incapacitated person has no willing and available family members or friends—hence, no private party to be appointed as guardian—and therefore is in real danger of falling between the cracks. In some places, private for-profit guardianship corporations, public guardianship agencies, or volunteer nonprofit guardianship programs may be available to accept judicial appointments when needed for these persons, especially if there is money involved. In their absence, though, important choices, including those pertaining to health care, may not be made until there is an emergency, and then consent to lifesaving treatment may be presumed as a matter of law. When that scenario unfolds, health care providers may end up functioning as unappointed patient surrogates, generally without any meaningful knowledge of the patient's own relevant wishes and values.

Another alternative to guardianship is the representative payee ("rep payee") system set up by federal law for handling government benefit checks (for example, those issued by the Social Security retirement or disability programs) on behalf of decisionally incapacitated beneficiaries. Appointment of a surrogate to receive and manage the payments is accomplished through a relatively simple administrative process. Many states have created a counterpart system for handling state benefit checks issued to incapacitated beneficiaries.

Cognitively impaired older persons also may come into contact with their locale's Adult Protective Services (APS) agency. Under a mandate of the Older Americans Act (42 United States Code § 3001), every state has set up an APS system to make available an array of social, medical, legal, and maintenance services to older non-institutionalized persons in need. Usually, older persons accept these services quite willingly, and the most pressing challenge for caregivers is obtaining enough resources to satisfy the individual's needs. Sometimes, however, individuals object to unwanted APS intrusions into their lives. State APS statutes usually contain provisions allowing for the forced imposition of services over the older person's objections in emergency circumstances, based on an abbreviated application and hearing process. Once the immediate emergency has abated, the APS agency must follow the normal guardianship process in that jurisdiction before proceeding with further intervention over the individual's protestations.

## AGE DISCRIMINATION

The Age Discrimination in Employment Act (ADEA) (29 United States Code § 621) was passed by Congress and signed into law in 1967 to protect people against discrimination in the work context based exclusively on their age. The ADEA, building on the Civil Rights Act of 1964, imposes on most private and public sector employers, employment agencies, and labor unions certain obligations to avoid discrimination (specifically, the responsibility to treat everyone equally regardless of age) in the areas of hiring, termination, promotion, training, and other terms and conditions of employment or retirement. The earlier widespread industry practice of mandatory retirement is now prohibited, and restrictions on employers' prerogative to offer early voluntary retirement ("buyout") plans were established by the 1990 federal Older Workers Benefit Protection Act and the 1991 amendments to the ADEA (29 United States Code § 626 [f]).

Under the ADEA, unequal treatment of particular workers or job applicants is permissible only on the basis of reasonable factors other than age (RFsOA), such as an individual's inability to perform the essential functions of the position satisfactorily, or in rare situations when age is a Bona Fide Occupational Qualification (BFOQ), as in piloting an airplane or working in public safety. Older workers who have been improperly discriminated against may have their rights enforced through a complaint to the Equal Employment Opportunity Commission

(EEOC) and ultimately through a civil action for money damages and injunctive relief (such as job reinstatement) brought in federal district court. Many states have enacted antidiscrimination statutes and have developed enforcement mechanisms that parallel those available at the federal level.

The ADEA additionally requires that any private insurance coverage that an employer chooses to offer its workers must be offered equally to workers over age 65. The employer's health plan is the primary payer, with Medicare paying eligible expenses that are not covered by the employer's plan. The reverse order of priority applies regarding private insurance coverage provided to an employer's retirees older than 65. The chief federal law affecting employee benefits, including health insurance, is the Employee Retirement and Income Security Act (ERISA) (29 United States Code §§ 1001 et seq.).

Older persons also may be protected against discrimination by the 1990 Americans with Disabilities Act (ADA) (42 United States Code § 12101 et seq.). That statute and its implementing regulations prohibit discrimination solely on account of disability in the work context (Title I), public services (Title II), and public accommodations (Title III) against individuals who have (or had previously or are considered by others to have) significant physical or mental diseases or defects that substantially impair their ability to perform major life activities. A sizable number of older persons would qualify for protection against discrimination under the ADA.

## CONCLUSION

The growth and recognition of the field of elder law as a distinct area of study and practice has profound implications for older individuals, families, gerontological professionals, and the larger society. Members of the elderly cohort are now well established as distinct subjects and consumers of legal activities, and individuals and agencies that serve older persons are very cognizant that they function within a particular legal environment. Laws and procedures that target the elderly for specific treatment, or that are generic on their face but contain special nuances when applied to older persons, are tools that both embody and help to create more sensitive social attitudes and respectful consideration of our aging compatriots.

## REFERENCES

American Bar Association. (1998). *Legal guide for older Americans: The law every American over fifty needs to know.* New York: Times Books.

Dayton, A. K., Gallanis, T. P., & Wood, M. M. (2003). *Elder law: Readings, cases, and materials* (2nd ed.). Cincinnati, OH: Anderson.

Frolik, L. A. (2002). The developing field of elder law redux: Ten years after. *Elder Law Journal, 10,* 1–5.

Frolik, L. A., & Barnes, A. P. (2003). *Elder law: Cases and materials* (3rd ed.). Dayton, OH: Lexis-Nexis.

Frolik, L. A., & Kaplan, R. L. (2003). *Elder law in a nutshell* (3rd ed.). St. Paul, MN: Est Group.

Kapp, M. B. (2001). *Lessons in law and aging: A tool for educators and students.* New York: Springer.

Kapp, M. B. (2002, Summer). Where will I live? How do housing choices get made for older persons? *NAELA Quarterly—Journal of the National Academy of Elder Law Attorneys, 15,* 2–5.

Mishkin, B., Mezey, M., & Ramsey, G. (1995). Advance directives in health care: Living wills and durable powers of attorney. In G. L. Maddox (Ed.), *The encyclopedia of aging* (2nd ed., pp. 26–28). New York: Springer.

Thomas, N., & Ingham, R. (2003). *State legal assistance development program study.* Available at www.tcsg.org/borchardstudy

Zimny, G. H., & Grossberg, G. T. (1998). *Guardianship of the elderly: Psychiatric and judicial aspects.* New York: Springer.

# 14

# Ethics and the Elderly

## *Eileen R. Chichin*

A lthough ethical issues confront us across the life span, they are most prominent when individuals are particularly vulnerable. Basic human rights belong to everyone, but for the dependent among us (e.g., infants, children, minorities, the frail elderly, etc.) they assume a greater magnitude. Advances in medical science and public health have resulted in a significant increase in life expectancy. In fact, the largest growing segment of the population in the United States is those over the age of 85. Many live the majority of their added years in relative good health, but at a certain point most will suffer from one or more chronic illness. Thus, there is a significant segment of our society that is burdened by frailty and increasing dependence.

This prospect causes concern for frail older persons, their families and friends, and society. It also presents us with a number of ethical issues. How we as a society address these issues is often a challenge to professionals working with a older population. As Jecker (1992, p. v) reminds,

> On one hand, as individuals, we grapple with the immediate experience of aging and mortality and seek to find in it philosophical or ethical significance. We also wonder what responsibilities we bear toward aging family members and what expectations of others our plans for old age can reasonably include. On the other hand, as a community, we must decide: what special role, if any, do older persons occupy in our society? What constitutes a just distribution of medical resources between generations? And how can institutions that serve the old foster imperiled values such as autonomy, self respect, and dignity? [p. v]

Care of older persons drives society to deal with ethics in the here and now and in an applied fashion. To do so in the most appropriate manner possible, gerontological professionals need a working knowledge of ethical principles and some framework for dealing with the sensitive ethical issues they regularly face. What happens as frail older persons face physical and cognitive decline affects them, their families, and society. At that time, ethical principles move out of the ivory tower and into the trenches.

This chapter addresses many of the ethical challenges that confront older persons and those who care for them, and attempts to provide some tools for resolution. Among the topics covered are respect for autonomy, the role of personal values, health care decision making, the allocation of resources, and the conflict between individual rights to self-determination and professional standards of care.

## WHAT DO WE MEAN BY ETHICS?

Various scholars use different terminology to define the term "ethics." A comprehensive description has been set forth by Fahey (1994) who describes ethics as "the systematic study of the appropriateness of human behavior . . . based on a perception of what it is to be human; in what human dignity consists; how society should function; and how humans should live within the context of the environment" (p. 5). The field of bioethics developed during the middle of the twentieth century as a result of several factors, to be described later in this chapter. The word "bioethics" evolved over time to become a term that is often used interchangeably with such others as medical ethics, nursing ethics, and health care ethics (Powers, 2003).

## KEY ETHICAL PRINCIPLES GUIDING THE CARE
## OF OLDER PEOPLE

There are three main ethical principles that should guide those involved with older persons: beneficence, autonomy, and justice. Each of these principles can stand alone; however they are often intertwined in practice.

### Beneficence

The first principle, beneficence, or doing good, clearly should guide all of our actions. The dilemma that often arises in health and social care settings when providers are attempting to provide care and services to older persons is that the desire of providers to do good is in direct opposition to what a client may wish for himself.

## Autonomy

The second principle, respect for autonomy, is generally considered the cornerstone of contemporary bioethics. Derived from the Greek for "self" and "rule," autonomy is so deeply entrenched in independence-loving American society that it was legislated in 1991 with the passage of the federal Patient Self-Determination Act (PSDA). This law assures each person of the right to accept or refuse treatment, even if refusing such treatment would result in death.

## Justice

Justice, the third governing principle, is also a key component of the American belief system and of particular import in decisions associated with how we allocate scarce resources. In writing about health and social care settings, Joseph Cardinal Bernadin (1985) emphasized our responsibility to the powerless among us, specifically, those that are old, young, hungry or homeless. How to do this, however, becomes a daunting challenge when the needs are great but the resources are limited.

## WHAT IS AN ETHICAL DILEMMA?

An ethical dilemma arises when there is some evidence that a particular act is morally right and some evidence that suggests it is morally wrong. Perhaps two of the more controversial ethical dilemmas in our society today are abortion and assisted suicide. With respect to older persons, however, a common "everyday" ethical dilemma is the case of a frail older community-dwelling woman living in the home she has lived in for 60 years. Her neighborhood is declining and becoming more dangerous, and she is becoming too functionally disabled to care for herself. Respecting her autonomy may dictate that her desire to remain in her home should be respected, but concern for her safety may find worried family members suggesting relocation. Whose values are more to be implemented? Which ethical principle should take precedence:

her family's concern for her safety (beneficence) or her desire to remain at home (respect for autonomy)?

Yet another common situation occurs when a health care team caring for a frail elderly patient believes strongly that the person will benefit by the use of sophisticated medical technology. Counter to the team's wishes, however, the patient refuses. The health care team is driven by beneficence (and to a great extent, by paternalism), but the patient's autonomy should take precedence.

## HISTORICAL EVENTS AND TRENDS INFLUENCING THE FIELD OF BIOETHICS

The need for the discipline of bioethics grew out of several factors. As noted earlier, advances in public health and medical technology allow us to live longer lives, but in an environment in which difficult choices often must be made.

New technologies such as cardiopulmonary resuscitation (CPR), feeding tubes, and hemodialysis were developed in the middle of the twentieth century. These technologies, when used appropriately, can extend life and improve its quality. There are instances, however, when decisions to use these technologies are counter to an individual's wishes or may cause more burden than benefit. The very existence of these technologies, however, often influence health care providers to suggest their use.

### Paternalism

The consumer movement of the 1970s also changed the way health care decisions are made. Prior to this, paternalism (the idea that doctors know best, and that they should make all health care decisions) was the dominant principle in health care. Thus, as a rule, decisions were made for patients by physicians with little or no patient input. Murphy (1984) illustrates this rather dramatically with her study of the moral reasoning of nurses. Exploring the views of nurses who were educated in the 1960s when they were socialized to the bottom of the health care pyramid, she found a significant number of these professionals expressing their primary loyalty to physicians and hospitals. When nurses were confronted with situations in which patients' rights and interests were pitted against those of the hospital or the doctor, they saw their primary responsibility to the physician and the institution.

The belief in medical paternalism began to be questioned in the 1960s and 1970s when different reform movements led to increased public scrutiny of health care institutions. Concomitantly, a number of medical research scandals involving physicians' experimentation on vulnerable populations such as indigent, elderly, African-American men and mentally retarded children fueled distrust of many in the medical profession (Steinbock, Arras, & London, 2003).

## Other Trends

An awareness of the limited number of health care resources (e.g., organs for transplantation) and decisions about rationing by age is another dilemma presented by a burgeoning older population. How much of the Medicaid dollar should be spent on nursing home care, and how much on, for example, younger women and children in poverty?

In addition, there is a growing consumer movement insisting upon truth telling in medicine and patients' rights to a basic level of health care, including the issue of who decides what constitutes "basic."

Court cases in the last decades of the twentieth century brought issues around one's right to die to the forefront. Although the more notorious cases involved young people (e.g., Karen Ann Quinlan and Nancy Cruzan [Ahronheim, Moreno, & Zuckerman, 2000]), they illustrate very dramatically the challenges associated with determining who makes health care decisions for those who are unable to do so for themselves—an issue particularly relevant in later life. The growing trend toward patient autonomy reached its peak in 1991 with the passage of the Patient Self Determination Act (PSDA). As a result of this legislation, all health care facilities and programs (i.e., hospitals, nursing homes, and home care programs) that receive federal funding are mandated to inform their patients and clients of their right to make health care decisions, including the right to accept or refuse any treatment. Inherent in this legislation is the recommendation that individuals execute an advance directive (living will, durable power of attorney for health care, or health care proxy) to ensure that their preferences about treatment will be known and respected in the event that illness or disability renders them unable to articulate these preferences.

The field of bioethics developed in response to these issues. Its body of knowledge gives guidance to lay persons and professionals in health and social care settings, emphasizing the utilization of ethical principles to address the dilemmas that arise in the everyday care of older persons as well as the more dramatic issues that accompany the end of life. It is imperative that human service professionals, particularly those who work with the frail elderly, have an awareness of the role of ethics and the application of ethical principles in their work with this vulnerable population.

## SOCIAL ISSUES AND ETHICS

Every culture believes that it has at least some responsibility for its aging population, although the degree to which filial responsibility is the norm varies from culture to culture. The gerontological literature supports the idea that most older people regard their families as their main social support system, and a considerable number of frail older persons reside near or with family members. When formerly independent older persons enter advanced old age and experience physical and cognitive decline, greater support from informal (family and friends) and formal (e.g., churches and synagogues, social service agencies, long-term care institutions) is needed.

As physical and cognitive decline increases, so do the ethical challenges. Balancing an elder's autonomy and safety demands a great deal of skill. When does an adult child strongly urge an aging, sunbelt-dwelling parent to relocate closer to the child? When does that child almost forcibly make that happen? What about the unsafe older driver? One of the more dramatic experiences for aging individuals living primarily in suburban and rural areas is the awareness, either by the individual or those close to him, of that person's loss of the ability to drive safely. A particularly difficult task for concerned families and often health care providers is informing the older person that he or she should no longer be behind the wheel. Increasingly, we are seeing advocacy groups for older persons (e.g., AARP) responding negatively when suggestions are made to arbitrarily limit driving privileges based on age. It is suggested that this is a form of limiting the autonomy of older persons. Nonetheless, it is likely that at some point states will pass legislation that requires driving and vision tests for persons of a certain age. In the meantime, physicians or families are often in the position of taking the car keys from older persons.

The majority of older persons reside in the community and strongly prefer to remain in that setting. As the social support literature reminds us, even very frail elders can continue to live at home with assistance from informal networks, formal programs, or a combination of both. Other older persons who remain functionally and cognitively capable of living alone may also continue to do so. Problems tend to arise when illness or advancing age causes safety issues to emerge. Older persons who reside with or very near family or who have access to health and social support programs may often remain in the community for many years. However, the group of individuals over 85—the oldest-old segment of our population—is growing faster than any other group. These individuals are most likely to suffer from debilitating conditions associated with advanced age, such as dementia and hip fractures. Thus, it is anticipated that decisions about institutionalization may arise with greater frequency. The dilemma described earlier in this chapter—the increasingly frail individual living in the unsafe home or neighborhood—may become more the norm. Accordingly, gerontological professionals will be confronted with the need to recommend and provide long-term care.

### Case Study: Mrs. Allen

*Mrs. Allen is an 86-year-old woman who lives in a large east coast city in a fourth-floor walk-up apartment. Widowed four years ago, she had lived with her husband in the same building since their marriage 63 years ago. Both her children lived in the apartment until they left home in their mid-twenties. Mrs. Allen's daughter lives in a suburb about half an hour from Mrs. Allen, and her son lives in California.*

*In relatively good health until her husband's death, Mrs. Allen has been slowly declining. Her gait is unsteady, and her daughter is concerned that her mother's memory is not what is used to be. In addition, the neighborhood seems to be falling into disrepair, and there has been some increase in crime in the area. Mrs. Allen's daughter has been asking Mrs. Allen to move in with her in the suburbs, but Mrs. Allen insists she is a city person and besides, this has always been her home.*

*One morning, Mrs. Allen's daughter is unable to reach her mother by telephone, and calls a neighbor to ask her to check. Upon entering Mrs. Allen's apartment, the neighbor finds her on the floor, where she had spent the night after tripping and falling in the kitchen. The neighbor calls Mrs. Allen's daughter and an ambulance, and Mrs. Allen is transported to the hospital, where her daughter meets her in the emergency room.*

## ETHICAL ISSUES IN INSTITUTIONAL SETTINGS

The institutional settings in which people are likely to spend time in their later years are the hospital and the nursing home. Although these two health care settings differ in many ways, they also have some issues in common. Most prominent in both settings is perhaps the need to make decisions about treatment.

As noted earlier, with the passage of the Patient Self Determination Act all adults are granted the right to accept or reject any health care treatment, even one that is necessary to stay alive. In the hospital setting, the acute nature of the illness and the treatment decisions that are made can make these decisions quite dramatic. An older individual may have been in relatively good health one day and then suffers a major heart attack or stroke the next. His family is suddenly faced with the need to make a life or death decision.

One treatment decision that older persons and their families are called on to make in acute care settings such as nursing homes, and even in the community is cardiopulmonary resuscitation (CPR). This procedure, which was developed to restart the heartbeat and breathing in situations in which one or both have stopped, has varying degrees of success. The success of CPR depends upon a number of factors, including how quickly after the event the procedure is begun, age, level of frailty, and underlying condition of the person who suffers a cardiopulmonary arrest. A person's ethical right to refuse CPR also has legal support in the DNR (do not resuscitate) law. Health care teams often suggest DNR when they believe the procedure will be ineffective. Decisions by individuals not to have CPR, based on DNR orders, are generally made when a person is ill or frail and wishes to end his or her days in a peaceful fashion. In fact, some health care facilities no longer use the negative term "DNR" but prefer the more positive "Allow Natural Death" ("AND").

Other decisions that hospitalized patients must make include diagnostic tests and surgery. If the older person is particularly frail, the outcome may be death, no matter what decision is made.

### Case Study: Mrs. Allen (continued)

*Mrs. Allen is admitted to the hospital from the emergency room and has surgery to repair her fractured hip. After surgery, because she is still sedated, the health care team asks her daughter about a "do not resuscitate" (DNR) order. The staff tell the daughter that this means only that they will not attempt to restart Mrs. Allen's heartbeat and breathing in the event these functions cease, and that she will receive all other medical treatment. Mrs. Allen's daughter tells the staff that she believes her mother would not want cardiopulmonary resuscitation to be attempted, and she agrees to a DNR order.*

*While Mrs. Allen is recovering in the hospital, a social worker talks to her about a durable power of attorney. Mrs. Allen decides it would be a wise idea to execute this advance directive, and with the social worker's assistance, she fills out the form and names her daughter to make health care decisions for her, should she become unable to do so. She tells the social worker she has complete confidence in her daughter, knowing that she would make whatever decisions she feels are in her mother's best interests.*

*Plans are made for Mrs. Allen to be transferred to a nursing home for short-term rehabilitation so that she will be able to function independently when she returns home. Mrs. Allen's daughter expresses some concern about her mother's ability to live alone in her old home, but wants to respect her mother's wishes regarding her living situation. Unfortunately, the day she is to be transferred she suffers a massive stroke and is completely unresponsive. She is maintained on intravenous hydration, but after another week in the hospital with no improvement whatsoever, the intravenous is stopped and Mrs. Allen is transferred to the nursing home.*

## LIVING IN A NURSING HOME

Although age and illness are not synonymous, there is the increasing likelihood of illness with advancing age. The more common scenario, however, is for older persons to live with chronic illness. At times, acute exacerbations of these conditions will be cause for hospitalization. As people grow older and frailer, they rarely return to the same baseline after being hospitalized. Conditions such as cardiovascular disease and cancer become much more common in later life, and with increasing age the incidence of dementia increases. Hip fractures occur with relative frequency, and often signal the beginning of a downhill slide. Thus, although a majority of older persons return home after hospitalization, at a certain point transfer to a long-term care facility is the more appropriate option. Others may enter a nursing home from the community, generally when social supports are unavailable or exhausted (Silin, 2001).

Because dependency is so feared, the thought of living in a nursing home may be one of the more frightening aspects of later life. Many adult children of institutionalized elders describe past conversations in which one or both parents stated emphatically, "Please don't ever put me in a nursing home!" Filial responsibility exists to varying degrees, and families do provide the bulk of care to frail elders. Nonetheless, often a time arises when a family's physical, emotional, and financial abilities are stretched to the limit and long-term institutional care is the only option. This is often after every available community-based service has been exhausted, and the caregiving family simply cannot continue to provide 24-hour care. Even in situations where the family realizes its limitations, and understands that the older individual is safer in an institutional environment, guilt—however irrational—still prevails, and may influence decisions that are made after admission to the home.

The nursing home setting is fraught with ethical concerns about the day-to-day issues as well as the more dramatic end-of-life issues. Institutional living in and of itself limits autonomy. Nursing home staff members at all levels face challenges to supporting the self-determination of their residents. Kane and Caplan (1990) describe many of the barriers to autonomy that those living in nursing homes encounter on a day-to-day basis. Admission to a nursing home is generally involuntary and often distressing to the individual and his or her loved ones. Although there are numerous efforts in many countries, including the United States, to change the institutional environment in nursing homes to more homelike settings through various "culture change" initiatives (Powers, 2003), for the most part nursing homes are markedly institutional in character. Regulations emphasize safety, and much of the day is routinized in a way that emphasizes staff rather than resident preferences. Thus, any semblance of autonomy on a day-to-day basis is difficult to find. As Kane and Caplan (1990) remind us: "Three enemies of personal autonomy for nursing home residents are: routine, regulation, and restricted opportunity" (p. 19). The dominant dilemmas in nursing home life, as perceived by those that live and work there, are not necessarily life and death issues. Rather, they are the more mundane, everyday issues of when and with whom one eats meals, awakens, and uses the telephone. While not as dramatic as issues associated with withholding or withdrawing life-sustaining treatment, they are based in autonomy nonetheless.

## HEALTH CARE DECISION MAKING IN THE NURSING HOME

Although many nursing home residents live in relatively stable health for many months to many years, acute illness may strike at any time. As well, increasing cognitive decline is common in this population. Accordingly, to ensure that an individual's preferences regarding treatment are known and respected, nursing home residents are encouraged to execute advance directives before they are limited by cognitive incapacity.

## Advance Directives

A number of older persons who enter a nursing home have completed some type of advance directive prior to entering the facility. Others who do not have directives may be suffering from dementia at the time of admission to the facility, but in some cases may still retain sufficient decision-making capacity to execute a durable power of attorney for health care or a health care proxy in states where those documents are the accepted advance directive. In states where living wills are the legal advance directives, the stage of dementia may preclude a nursing home resident's ability to execute such a document. (The execution of a living will requires that the person executing it have the ability to make decisions about specific treatments, whereas to execute a durable power of attorney, the individual only has to be able to appoint someone to make decisions.) This is added support for encouraging adults of all ages to make treatment wishes known in advance of disability.

## The Absence of Advance Directives

In the absence of an advance directive, treatment for those who are unable to make their own decisions should be consistent with what the individual would have wanted, to the greatest degree possible. This generally requires an in-depth discussion of the individual's treatment wishes, if known, and personal values, including religious beliefs. Health care decision making for persons without decision-making capacity and without advance directives who have no one to speak for them—referred to as the unbefriended elderly—is perhaps the most challenging situation. In these cases the nursing home is obligated to provide treatment unless the medical team believes doing so would be futile or inordinately burdensome.

## Making Treatment Decisions

As noted earlier, the Patient Self Determination Act mandates that all health care institutions that receive Medicare or Medicaid funding inform their patients regarding their rights to make any and all treatment decisions. Many health care professionals believe the work in this area is done when a person executes an advance directive. Optimally, however, this should only be the first step in health care decision making in the nursing home; health care decision making is best viewed as a process.

One can generally anticipate that decisions about certain treatments will arise during a nursing home stay. To prevent crisis management, it is wise for health care professionals in long-term care settings to learn, in advance of a resident's decline, what his or her preferences for treatment are. The decisions that most often must be made include questions of resuscitation, artificial nutrition and hydration, intravenous antibiotics, and the use of diagnostic tests (Carter & Chichin, 2003).

## Resuscitation Decisions

The issue of attempting resuscitation versus an order not to resuscitate (DNR order) should be discussed with all nursing home residents or their responsible relatives/friends. The procedure itself, as well as its pros and cons, should be described. Of note is that the success rate of cardiopulmonary resuscitation in frail nursing home patients is extremely poor (Kane & Burns, 1997). Family members are often reluctant to agree to a DNR order because they feel they are signing a death warrant. The reality is, however, that only a tiny percentage of nursing home patients will survive this procedure.

Another issue with respect to a "do not resuscitate order" is that it only pertains to attempts to restart the heartbeat and breathing in cases where these activities have stopped; it does not preclude the provision of any other treatment.

## Hospitalization Decisions

A second treatment decision that should be discussed is hospitalization. Specifically, if acute illness occurs, would the resident want to be kept in the nursing home and kept as comfortable as possible, or would he or she wish to be sent to an acute care hospital? Often, early in a person's nursing home stay, if the individual is relatively well, hospitalization for some situations may be appropriate. In other cases, however, where physical and cognitive decline are significant or where there have been a number of hospitalizations in the past, consideration might be given to not hospitalizing again. Transfer to a hospital is distressing to a nursing home resident at best, and if the frail older person returns to the nursing home, it is generally at a lower baseline than when he or she left it. Perhaps most important, it should be emphasized that a decision not to hospitalize does not mean that solid medical and nursing care, including pain management, will not be provided in the nursing home (Carter & Chichin, 2003).

## Diagnostic Testing Decisions

Other decisions related to treatment have to do with the use of diagnostic tests. Many of these procedures, including electrocardiograms, x-rays, and blood tests may be useful and appropriate early in some nursing home stays. As a person declines over time, however, thought should be given to whether these procedures are of sufficient benefit to perform them or whether they will be burdensome to the resident. Additionally, there may come a time when there is no need to perform diagnostic tests because nothing will be done with the results.

## Medication Decisions

The use of intravenous antibiotics is another decision that should be considered. Nursing home residents are prone to developing infections, and although oral antibiotics are often used, occasionally intravenous antibiotics are suggested. Residents and families may request that this procedure be avoided if the burdens associated with it (e.g., repeated needle sticks, etc.) outweigh the benefits (Carter & Chichin, 2003).

## Artificial Nutrition and Hydration Decisions

A very common decision that needs to be made in the nursing home setting involves the use of artificial nutrition and hydration. This is one of the most difficult decisions for loved ones to make, essentially because of the tendency to associate food with love and nurturing. The idea of not using artificial nutrition conjures up thoughts of someone "starving to death." However, there is a growing literature that suggests that individuals near the end of life are more comfortable without artificial food and fluids (Ahronheim, 1996; Finucane, Christmas, & Travis, 1999; Gillick, 2000; McCann, Hall, & Groth-Juncker, 1994). Thus, if comfort is the main goal for a person at the end of life, the use of artificial nutrition and hydration should generally be avoided.


## The Resident's Wishes

For all the treatment decisions described above, the key factor that should guide decision-making is the individual resident's wishes, if these are known. If they are not known to the health care team and to the involved family, decisions should be made in what is considered to be in the individual's best interest. It should be noted that determining the goals of care for the individual should guide decision making. If comfort is the primary goal, then decisions about particular treatments should be made in a way that will achieve comfort. This generally involves, at least near the end of life, minimizing the use of medical technologies and maximizing the use of any interventions that enhance comfort and dignity. These interventions may include medications to treat uncomfortable symptoms, as well as providing a de-medicalized environment that includes natural lighting, quiet or soft music, and such low-tech things as hand holding and talking to the patient.

### Case Study: Mrs. Allen (continued)

*After admitting Mrs. Allen to the nursing home, the health care team meets with her daughter to discuss a plan of care. Mrs. Allen's daughter is very tearful as she tells the team that her mother was a very independent person and would never want to have her life extended by the use of tubes of any kind. The team tells the daughter that Mrs. Allen will most likely pass away within a few days to a few weeks without any fluids or nourishment. The daughter says she understands that, but feels obligated to respect her mother's values. The team promises to do everything possible to keep Mrs. Allen (and her daughter) comfortable so that Mrs. Allen's final days will be spent in peace and dignity and her daughter will have the memory of her mother's having what many would refer to as a "good death."*

Caring for the frail elderly, especially nursing home patients at the end of life, is an ethical challenge today because the wide variety of life-sustaining technologies exist in an era where respect for patient autonomy (and therefore, respect for their wishes when known) is dominant. Gerontological professionals can be guided by the words of Quill and McCann (2003):

Those who care for incapacitated patients have an important and difficult job. These patients are vulnerable and sick and cannot speak for themselves. The medical task is to enhance the quality and meaning of their lives and to try to give them a central voice in balancing disease-driven and palliative treatments by keeping what is known about their values and wishes at the center of clinical decision-making. Alleviating discomfort and avoiding harm are imperative. It is a challenging and uncertain process, so every effort should be made to achieve a consensus among those who care about the patient on the proper course of action. . . . Our severely ill, incapacitated patients are counting on us not to walk away from this challenge. [p. 340]

## ETHICAL ISSUES FACING SOCIETY

Care of the frail older population in general is a daunting task for society. The primary concerns center on the cost of care and the allocation of resources. A number of philosophers and politicians in the past few decades have debated the issue of age as it relates to health care resources. One of the first of these was Callahan (1987), who argued in his book, *Setting Limits*, that health care should be rationed by age. A few years later, Governor Richard Lamm of Colorado also agreed with this premise (Moody, 2002).

At present, people over 65 in this country account for about one-third of all national health care expenses (Moody, 2002). As our population is growing older, it seems likely that more people will question the degree to which this kind of spending should continue. The reality is that rationing does occur in subtle ways. When a 35-year-old and an 85-year-old with similar illnesses are vying for the remaining ICU bed, to whom will the health care facility give that bed?

Although the aging of the population is not the sole factor influencing increased health care costs, it works in concert with increases in services, utilization rates, new technologies, and higher wages for health care workers (Moody, 2002). This problem will continue to confront our society, and clearly some creative approaches to these issues must be sought.

## SUMMARY AND CONCLUSION

Numerous ethical issues affect older persons, their families, and the gerontological professionals who serve them. These issues range from such basic, seemingly mundane decisions such as taking the car keys away from a parent or grandparent, to the more complex concerns associated with ensuring comfort and dignity in that parent or grandparent's final days. Those who work with an older population owe it to their patients and clients to be knowledgeable about how to best address these issues. An awareness of the ethical components of the work we do is the first step.

## REFERENCES

Ahronheim, J. C. (1996). Nutrition and hydration in the terminal patient. *Clinics of Geriatric Medicine, 12,* 379–391.

Ahronheim, J. C., Moreno, J. D., & Zuckerman, C. (2000). *Ethics in clinical practice* (2nd ed.). Gaithersburg, MD: Aspen.

Bernadin, J. (1985). Health care and the consistent ethic of life. *Origins, 15*(3), 36–40.

Carter, J. M., & Chichin, E. R. (2003). Palliative care in the nursing home. In R. S. Morrison & D. E. Meier (Eds.), *Geriatric palliative care* (pp. 357–375). New York: Oxford University Press.

Fahey, C. (1994). The moral aspects of the Patient Self-Determination Act. In M. B. Kapp (Ed.), *Patient self-determination in long-term care* (pp. 1–10). New York: Springer.

Finucane, T. E., Christmas, M., & Travis, K. (1999). Tube feeding in patients with advanced dementia: A review of the evidence. *Journal of the American Medical Association, 282,* 1365–1370.

Gillick, M. (2000). Rethinking the role of tube feeding in patients with advanced dementia. *New England Journal of Medicine, 342,* 206–210.

Jecker, N. (1992). *Aging and ethics.* Totowa, NJ: Humana.

Kane, R. A., & Caplan, A. L. (Eds.). (1990). *Everyday ethics: Resolving dilemmas in nursing home life.* New York: Springer.

Kane, R. S., & Burns, E. A. (1997). Cardiopulmonary resuscitation policies in long-term care facilities. *Journal of the American Geriatric Society, 45,* 154–157.

McCann, R. M., Hall, W. J., & Groth-Juncker, A. (1994). Comfort care for terminally ill patients: The appropriate use of nutrition and hydration. *Journal of the American Medical Association, 272,* 1263–1266.

Murphy, C. P. (1984, September). The changing role of nurses in making ethical decisions. *Law, Medicine and Health Care, 12,* 173–175, 184.

Powers, B. (2003). *Nursing home ethics.* New York: Springer.

Quill, T. E., & McCann, R. (2003). Decision-making for the cognitively impaired. In R. S. Morrison & D. E. Meier (Eds.), *Geriatric palliative care* (pp. 332–341). New York: Oxford University Press.

Silin, P. S. (2001). *Nursing homes: The family's journey.* Baltimore: Johns Hopkins University Press.

Steinbock, B., Arras, J. D., & London, A. J. (2003). *Ethical issues in modern medicine* (6th ed.). New York: McGraw-Hill.

# 15

# Identifying and Preventing Elder Abuse

## Thomas M. Cassidy

I t is not uncommon for people to associate elder abuse with a frightening news report of a patient being abused in a nursing home. However, the overwhelming majority of elder abuse incidents are much more subtle and occur when older people are physically, emotionally, or psychologically abused in the home. As a group, people 65 and older are less likely to be victims of violent crime than younger men and women (Klaus, 2000). However, it is estimated that each year more than two million older Americans are victims of elder abuse, neglect, and financial exploitation, and that number may be significantly higher as many cases are not reported (American Psychological Association, 2003).

When a patient is abused in a nursing home, there are safeguards in place to detect and correct the problem. In addition to shifts of workers who provide direct and supervisory care for patients, government regulators conduct routine announced and unannounced inspections of nursing homes to ensure that patients are receiving appropriate care. Although not perfect, these safeguards are effective. There are no such safeguards in the home, especially when the abuse is a continuation of a family pattern that has been occurring for many years. For example, there are no routine interventions or inspections to assist an elderly woman who has tolerated abusive behavior during many years of marriage, or an elderly parent who is dependent on an adult child with an alcohol or substance abuse problem or a personality disorder. Social isolation is a risk factor for elder abuse and can also be a clue that a family or an individual is in trouble (APA, 2003).

## THE NATIONAL CENTER ON ELDER ABUSE (NCEA)

The National Center on Elder Abuse, a national resource center for elder rights supported by the United States Administration on Aging, identifies the seven major types of elder abuse (NCEA, 2004). They are as follows:

1.  *Physical Abuse:* Physical abuse is the use of physical force that may result in bodily injury, physical pain, or impairment. It may include, but is not limited to, such acts of violence as striking (with or without an object), hitting, beating, pushing, shoving, shaking, slapping, kicking, pinching, and burning. Inappropriate use of drugs and physical restraints, force-feeding, and physical punishment of any kind also are examples of physical abuse. Signs and symptoms of physical abuse include bruises, black eyes, welts, lacerations, rope marks, and bone fractures. An elder's sudden change in behavior and the caregiver's refusal to allow visitors to see an elder alone should be investigated.

2.  *Sexual Abuse:* Sexual abuse is nonconsensual sexual contact of any kind with an elderly person. Sexual contact with any person incapable of giving consent is also considered sexual abuse. It includes, but is not limited to, unwanted touching and all types of sexual assault or battery, such as rape, sodomy, coerced nudity, and sexually explicit photographing.

3.  *Emotional or Psychological Abuse:* Emotional or psychological abuse is the infliction of anguish, pain, or distress through verbal or nonverbal acts. It includes, but is not limited to, verbal assaults, insults, threats, intimidation, humiliation, and harassment. In addition, treating an older person like an infant; isolating an elderly person from family, friends, or regular activities; and giving an older person the "silent treatment" are examples of emotional/psychological abuse.

4.  *Neglect:* Neglect is the refusal or failure to fulfill any part of a person's obligations or duties to an elder. It may also include failure of a person who has fiduciary responsibilities to provide care for an elder (i.e., pay for necessary home care services) or the failure on the part of an in-home service provider to provide necessary care. Neglect typically means the refusal or failure to provide an elderly person with such life necessities as food, water, clothing, shelter, personal hygiene, medicine, comfort, personal safety, and other essentials included in an implied or agreed-upon responsibility to an elder.

5.  *Abandonment:* Abandonment of the elderly is the desertion of an elderly person by an individual who has assumed responsibility for

providing care for an elder, or by a person with physical custody of an elder. Frail elderly patients have been deserted by their caregivers at hospitals, nursing facilities, and public locations.

6. *Financial or Material Exploitation:* Financial or material exploitation is the illegal or improper use of an elder's funds, property, or assets. Examples include, but are not limited to, cashing an elderly person's checks without authorization or permission; forging an older person's signature; misusing or stealing an older person's money or possessions; coercing or deceiving an older person into signing any document (e.g., contracts or will); and the improper use of conservatorship, guardianship, or power of attorney.

7. *Self-Neglect:* Self-neglect is the behavior of an elderly person that threatens his or her own health or safety. It generally manifests as a refusal or failure to provide himself or herself with adequate food, water, clothing, shelter, personal hygiene, medication (when indicated), and safety precautions. Self-neglect excludes a situation in which a mentally competent older person, who understands the consequences of his or her decisions, makes a conscious and voluntary decision to engage in acts that threaten his or her health or safety as a matter of personal choice.


## THE NATIONAL ELDER ABUSE INCIDENCE STUDY

The National Elder Abuse Incidence Study, released in 1998, was prepared for the Administration on Aging and the Administration for Children and Families (Tatara, 1998). This study, requested by Congress, confirmed what experts long believed, that reported cases of elder abuse are only the tip of the iceberg. This study estimates that for every incident of elder abuse that is reported, approximately five go unreported. This study also found that

- female elders are abused at a higher rate than males, after adjusting for their larger proportion in the aging population
- elders 80 years and older are abused and neglected at two to three times their proportion of the elderly population
- victims of self-neglect are usually depressed, confused, or extremely frail
- in almost 90% of elder abuse and neglect incidents with a known perpetrator, the perpetrator is a family member, and two-thirds of the perpetrators are adult children or spouses.

## REPORTING ELDER ABUSE

Family members of victims (20%), hospitals (17%), and police (11%) are the major reporters of substantiated cases of domestic elder abuse and neglect. The elder victims themselves report these incidents less than ten percent of the time. Physicians, nurses, and clinics each accounted for slightly less than ten percent of the substantiated domestic elder abuse reports (Tatara, 1998).

Because the majority of older people spend their later years in relatively good health and are not victims of elder crimes and abuses, people are sometimes caught off guard when they suspect that an elderly relative, friend, or patient has been the victim of elder abuse. This is especially true if the alleged victim is not complaining or cooperating. The Administration on Aging funded a study by the National Committee for the Prevention of Elder Abuse to teach professionals and the public how to identify and report elder abuse. The resulting publication, *Multidisciplinary Elder Abuse Prevention Teams* (Nerenberg, 2003), provides a guide to agencies and communities that use a team approach to coordinate resources when investigating elder abuse.

It is not the responsibility of health professionals and the public to investigate elder abuse, but rather it is their responsibility to report suspicions to those who are trained and mandated to investigate whether an incident is an accident, oversight, self-neglect, or abuse. One phone call, email, or letter could save an older victim from pain, suffering, and even death.

### Who Investigates Elder Abuse?

Every state has an elder abuse hotline to an agency or agencies that receive and investigate allegations of elder abuse. However, when an older person is in imminent danger, has been assaulted or abused, the police should be called immediately. In other circumstances, caseworkers at adult protective services (APS) are generally the designated first responders to reports of abuse (National Center on Elder Abuse, 2004b).

Because each state has its own elder abuse hotline phone numbers, a quick and easy way to find the hotline number in any state is to call the nationwide toll-free Eldercare Locator Service at 1-800-677-1116. This service, provided by the Administration on Aging, is designed to put people in touch with state and local resources (including the elder abuse hotline) available to assist the older American. The Eldercare

Locator is especially helpful for those who provide long-distance elder care.

## Resources for Reporting Elder Abuse

Adult Protective Services (APS) is the principal public agency responsible for investigating reported cases of elder and vulnerable adult abuse and for providing victims with treatment and protective services. A vulnerable adult is defined as a person who is being mistreated or is in danger of mistreatment and who, due to age and/or disability, is unable to protect him- or herself. If the investigators find abuse or neglect, they arrange for services to help protect the victim (NCEA, 2004b).

Other agencies responsible for investigating reported cases of elder abuse include police and sheriff departments, offices for the aging, long-term care ombudsman services, and the State Attorney General's Medicaid Fraud Control Unit.

## Write It Down

A written record of an alleged elder abuse incident is very helpful. It should include the date, time, and place that the incident occurred and the names of any witnesses and their observations. For example, consider the value of the following information when provided to an investigator or caseworker (Cassidy, 2004):

Date: _____ Time: _____ Place: _____

Name of Complainant: _____

Address: _____

Phone Number: _____

Name of Elder: _____ Age: ____ Date of Birth: ____

Address: _____

Phone Number: _____ Status of Patient: _____

Type of Possible Abuse: _____

Date of Occurrence/Observation: _____

Description of Complaint: _____

_____

Date and Location of Photographs or Videotapes: _____

Name and Description of Alleged Perpetrator: _____

_____

Names/Descriptions of Witnesses: _____

_____

Next of Kin or Authorized Person Notified: _____
Date: _____


## Caregiver Risks

All people are encouraged and many health care professionals are
required by law to report any suspicions of elder abuse as soon as
possible. Health professionals must address the needs of their patients
first and foremost, even under difficult circumstances. Exhausted and
overworked caregivers place their patients, jobs, licenses, and themselves
at great risk.

### Case Study 1

*An overworked medication nurse at a nursing home became the subject of
a patient neglect investigation when a health investigator, on a routine
inspection, observed that she neglected to dispense a prescribed drug to one
of her patients on several consecutive days. Fortunately in this case, there
was no apparent adverse reaction for the patient. This nurse attempted to
complete her rounds, but patient after patient asked her for some form of
comfort or for bathroom assistance, when her assignment was only to
dispense medications. With a finite period in which to complete her rounds,
whenever she took time to help a patient, another would be shortchanged
by that same amount of time. One of the last patients on her assigned list
required one of her medications within two hours of eating. On several
consecutive days, the medication nurse failed to reach that patient within
that time frame and therefore could not dispense needed medications.*

*Older patients often have multiple illnesses that require daily or several-
times-daily attention. This makes it difficult, if not impossible, to develop
a one-size-fits-all formula for staffing needs.*


## The Aggressive Patient

Although the great majority of older patients are cooperative and appreciative, some are not. Incidents of elder abuse sometimes occur in a

moment of anger or frustration, prompted by a confused patient's act of aggression. Health care professionals are trained to react calmly and to expect that some patients who suffer from dementia may yell, scream, curse, insult, and even attempt to kick or slap those who are trying to care for them. Those who are not properly trained put their patients and themselves at risk.

### Case Study 2

*A health aide on a morning shift was expecting to follow his routine assignment. He entered the bedroom expecting to change his patient's adult diaper, clean and dress him, then transfer him to his wheelchair and bring him to breakfast. The 89-year-old patient was daydreaming when he was approached by the aide. Startled, and embarrassed that he had wet his bed, the patient cursed, screamed a racial insult, and then struck the aide, who shoved the patient back into his bed, painfully bruising his chest. Later that day, when an investigator attempted to ask the patient how his chest was bruised, the patient described his pain using obscene language with ethnic and racial insults, groped the nurse who was standing by his wheelchair, and ended the interview abruptly, explaining that he had to get ready to go to work.*

## Family Caregivers

Many family caregivers are at risk for exhaustion. They often devote themselves so fully to their elder parent or spouse that they may neglect their own needs. Caregiver stress is a significant risk factor for abuse and neglect, especially if the caregiver has no skills for managing difficult behaviors. Sometimes, a well spouse or adult child is pressured into providing sole care for a chronically ill spouse or parent. This can cause tremendous physical, psychological, and emotional stress for the patient and the caregiver.

### Case Study 3

*An adult daughter was pressured by her frail and dying mother to be her sole caregiver. The daughter, who had built a successful business, suggested that she could hire a trained home health aide to care for her mother during the day, and she herself would provide care in the evenings and on the weekends. The mother refused this offer and told her daughter that she would only accept care from her. The daughter complied with her mother's*

*request and became a full-time caregiver for the rest of her mother's life,
which turned out to be six months. The responsibility of caring for a dying
patient without any training or respite care was the primary cause of the
daughter's being admitted to the hospital for depression shortly after her
mother's death. The unintended consequence of agreeing to accommodate
an unreasonable elder care demand is the potential for caregiver abuse.
In this case there was no physical abuse to either party, but both the elderly
mother and the adult daughter suffered a severe emotional and psychological
toll that could have been reduced or avoided with early planning and
professional help.*

## False Accusations

When a disoriented or confused elder cannot find a lost or misplaced
item he or she may falsely accuse caregivers or visitors of theft. When
items are actually stolen, the wrong person might be accused of theft.
For example, a nursing student who worked as a home health aide was
falsely accused of stealing checks from her elderly client. In this case,
the real thief, a neighbor, was arrested and prosecuted because the
bank had videotaped the transaction when she cashed the forged checks.

Those who provide care at home should be attentive to their patients
and observant of their surroundings. If they notice that cash, jewelry,
financial records, checkbooks, credit cards, or other valuables are visible
and unattended during their visits, it is important to recommend that
those items be put in a safe place, and then make an entry in their
patient's chart.

## THE LINK BETWEEN ELDER COSTS AND ELDER ABUSE

Medicare, the health insurer for the older population, does not pay for
long term-care, either in a nursing home or at home. When elderly
patients are about to be discharged from the hospital they often face
the prospect of having to pay the total cost of hiring home care workers
or paying for nursing home care. Such care is expensive and can easily
cost $50,000 per year or more. This unexpected stress has led many
Americans who have planned poorly or not at all for this expense to
use poor judgment and place an elder patient in the care of unlicensed
caregivers (Cassidy, 2004).

The risk of unnecessary pain, suffering, and even death for their
loved ones increases dramatically for those who hire from the under-

ground pool of unlicensed caregivers. Tragically, some patients and families would rather risk substandard care than pay for licensed and authorized care.

### Case Study 4

*An elderly mother with dementia, who was not poor enough to qualify for Medicaid (the health insurer for the poor), was placed in the care of an unlicensed caregiver by her adult children in order to save their inheritance. Slowly and painfully over a period of time the mother lost weight and eventually died of starvation. After her death, witnesses recalled watching this elderly woman devour a gift of ice cream and then start to eat the cardboard container, but no one called the police or the elder abuse hotline. It is truly tragic for elders when greed comes before need.*

## Untrained Caregivers

An elderly patient who fell and fractured her hip when her daughter attempted to move her from her bed to the bathroom provides a valuable lesson for all caregivers. As the mother started to slip toward the floor, she and her daughter screamed for help, but unfortunately it was too late. A fall can cause serious injury and may force an older person into a chronic or permanent need for a higher level of care, such as a hospital or nursing home. The Centers for Disease Control reports that in 2001 more than 1.6 million seniors were treated in emergency departments for fall-related injuries and more than 370,000 were hospitalized (NCIPC, 2003). In the above case, the daughter had no training as a caregiver and she thought she could handle the situation herself.

## ELDER FRAUD: AN EMERGING ISSUE

As the population ages, accumulates more wealth, and becomes more dependent on others, the conditions for fraud will ripen (Cassidy, 2004). The median net worth of households headed by those 65 and older increased by 69% between 1984 and 1999, whereas the median net worth for households headed by persons ages 45 to 54 declined by 23% during the same period. Older Americans are now the wealthiest segment of the population (Federal Forum on Aging Related Statistics,

2000). Those who commit fraud commonly target people with assets and take advantage of their position of trust.

Research has shown that people are more likely to fall for a scheme they have never heard about (Murray, 1999). With that in mind, it is helpful to look at some of the specific types of fraud schemes that target the older population.

## Telemarketing Fraud

Not all elder frauds are committed in the home. It is estimated that telemarketing fraud robs Americans of more than $40 billion annually. AARP (2002) found that 56% of the names of victims on "mooch lists" (what fraudulent telemarketers call their lists of most likely victims) were age 50 or older. The FBI estimates that about 14,000 illegal telemarketing operations are bilking consumers every day.

Older people are often the target of these operations partly because many elders believe that it is impolite to hang up on a caller. One way to reduce the possibility of being a victim of a telemarketing fraud is to have your phone number placed on the "do-not-call" registry at the state and federal level. The Federal Trade Commission (FTC) allows consumers to register their phone numbers on a national "do-not-call" registry at www.donotcall.gov or by calling 1-888-382-1222 (FTC, 2004a). It is illegal for most telemarketers to call a number listed on the registry.

## Internet Fraud

The Internet is another place where older consumers are at risk for fraud and deception. For example, health frauds may claim to provide "miracle" products and treatments that cure serious illness and are not sold through traditional suppliers. The FBI reports that the proportion of individuals losing at least $5,000 in Internet fraud is higher for victims 60 years of age and older than it is for any other age category (FBI, 2002).

## Identity Theft and Financial Fraud

Although electronic banking and credit cards are convenient, they also offer opportunities for fraud. Shredding junk mail such as preapproved credit card mailings and any financial records before they are put in the trash can stop thieves who steal identities by sorting through garbage and dumpsters. However, all consumers must understand that no matter how well they protect their mail, telephone, and Internet use, they are still at risk for identity theft. For example, consider the arrest of a software employee who stole the credit histories of 30,000 people and sold them to a ring of thieves. It could take days, months, or years before some of these victims become aware that their identities have been stolen (Cassidy, 2004). If an individual suspects that his or her identity has been stolen, The FTC (2004b) recommends taking the following four steps:

1.  Contact the fraud departments of any one of the three major credit bureaus (Equifax, Experian, and TransUnion) to place an alert on your credit file.
2.  Close the accounts that you suspect have been tampered with or opened fraudulently.
3.  File a police report.
4.  File a complaint with the FTC by contacting www.consumer.gov/ idtheft or contact the FTC's Identity Theft Hotline toll-free at 1-877-IDTHEFT (438-4338).

## Home Improvement Fraud

Fraudulent home improvement contractors often target older consumers because the elderly have a greater need for home improvements. They tend to live in older homes that need repair and they are less likely to do repairs themselves. It is important for older consumers to choose the right contractor for any repair or home improvement. An important first step is to get some recommendations, along with proof that the contractor is licensed, bonded, and covered by workers' compensation and liability insurance. It is wise to make a list of the specific things necessary for a contractor to repair or maintain. As a general rule, the more the consumers know at the beginning of a project, the better off they will be when the project ends (Hermanson & Moag, 1999).

## Investment Fraud

Retirees who are frightened about meeting their future income needs are especially vulnerable to get-rich-quick schemes. Often these scams are the work of unlicensed agents who lure older investors with "sure bets." It is always important to make certain that the person selling an investment is licensed, but don't stop there. Older consumers should never let anyone, whether licensed or not, pressure or scare them into making a quick decision.

## CONCLUSION

The risk of elder abuse, neglect, and financial exploitation can be drastically reduced when older people address difficult family, social, financial, and legal relationships with a team of those trained to help them. However, even those with the best of relationships and plans cannot eliminate all of the risks when cognitive illness strikes. A survey by the American Prosecutors Research Institute found that the diminished mental capacity of the victim was the most troublesome aspect of prosecuting elder abuse cases (Miller & Johnson, 2003).

In concluding this chapter, it is worthwhile to remember the words intended to be part of the last speech of President John Fitzgerald Kennedy, a speech that he was to deliver at a luncheon at the Dallas Trade Mart on November 22, 1963, the day of his death (Kennedy, 1963). He was assassinated only minutes before his scheduled talk: "We in this country, in this generation, are, by destiny rather than choice, the watchmen. . . . " Those who address the needs of the older population are often the last line of defense for the frail elderly. We must all be the watchmen!

## REFERENCES

American Association of Retired Persons. (2002). *Facts about fraudulent telemarketing.* Washington, DC: Author.
American Psychological Association. (2003). *Elder abuse and neglect: In search of solutions.* Washington, DC: Author. Available at www.apa.org
Cassidy, T. (1997). Home care fraud: The emerging epidemic. *The White Paper.* Austin, TX: Association of Certified Fraud Examiners.
Cassidy, T. (2004). *Elder care: What to look for, what to look out for!* Far Hills, NJ: New Horizon.
Federal Bureau of Investigation. (2002). *2001 Internet fraud report.* Washington, DC: U.S. Department of Justice.
Federal Forum on Aging Related Statistics. (2000). Older Americans 2000: Key Indicators of well-being. Hyattsville, MD: National Center for Health Statistics. Also available at www.agingstats.gov
Federal Trade Commission. (2004a). *National Do Not Call Registry.* Washington, DC: Author.

Federal Trade Commission. (2004b). *ID theft: When bad things happen to your good name*. Washington, DC: Author.

Hermanson, S., & Moag, K. (1999). *Home improvement contractors*. Washington, DC: American Association of Retired Persons.

Kennedy, J. F. (1963). *Remarks prepared for delivery at the Trade Mart in Dallas*. Columbia Point-Boston, MA: The John Fitzgerald Kennedy Library.

Klaus, P. (2000). *Crimes against persons age 65 or older, 1992–1997*. Washington, DC: U.S. Department of Justice.

Kochera, A. (2002). *Falls among older persons and the role of the home: An analysis of cost, incidence, and potential savings for home modification*. Washington, DC: American Association of Retired Persons.

Miller, M., & Johnson, J. (2003). Protecting America's senior citizens: What local prosecutors are doing to fight elder abuse. *Special Topic Series*, Sept. 2003, page 30. Alexandria, VA: American Prosecutors Research Institute.

Murray, C. (1999). How to avoid financial fraud. *Economic Education Bulletin*. Great Barrington, MA: American Institute for Economic Research. Vol. 39, #4, page 2.

National Center on Elder Abuse. (2004a). *The basics*. Available at www.elderabusecenter.org

National Center on Elder Abuse. (2004b). *Help for elders and families: Adult protective services*. Available at www.elderabusecenter.org

National Center on Elder Abuse Newsletter. (2003, December). *The top five most difficult aspects of prosecuting elder abuse cases*. Available at www.elderabusecenter.org

National Center for Injury Prevention and Control. (2003). *Falls and hip fractures among older adults*. Available at www.cdc.gov/ncipc

Nerenberg, L. (2003). *Multidisciplinary elder abuse prevention teams*. Washington, DC: National Center on Elder Abuse.

Tatara, T. (1998). *The national elder abuse incidence study*. Washington, DC: Administration on Aging, National Center on Elder Abuse. www/agingstats.gov

# 16

# Interdisciplinary Teamwork: The Key to Quality Care for Older Adults

## *Patricia A. Miller*

Why teamwork? It is well understood that advances in medical science and technology have contributed to the aging of the world's population. Chronic and multiple diseases and disability, prevalent in those living to advanced ages, often reduce independence, limit function in the activities and roles important to older adults, and require formal support services in and out of the institution. Therefore, it should be clear that one discipline alone cannot meet the multiple and complex needs older adults struggle with in their daily lives. Yet, despite the fact that teams are ubiquitous in health care, very few graduate educational programs provide courses that prepare practitioners for the role of team member or team leader. In fact, one might speculate that the development of a specialized body of knowledge and a professional identity, integral components of all graduate education, might inadvertently foster a chauvinistic attitude of novice practitioners, that is, "I can do it all!" Very soon, some graduates realize that they cannot do it all, and they either become disillusioned with the field of aging and move on to other areas of practice, or they learn to function as team members/leaders, working collaboratively with other disciplines to meet the dynamic challenges facing older adults and their caregivers.

This chapter is designed to prepare students and practitioners in the field of aging with the requisite tools to become effective team members and team leaders in order to provide coordinated, comprehensive, and quality care. The three basic concepts of team development, team management, and team process will be described. Examples will be drawn from the field of aging, illustrating the value of collaborative teamwork to the individuals we serve, to the community, and to society at large.

## THE PROS AND CONS OF TEAMWORK

The author does not want to imply that teams are the only means to quality care. Teams do not replace one-to-one interventions. Within this more intimate dynamic, practitioners have an opportunity to demonstrate to their clients a depth of caring and understanding of their needs, wishes, and priorities, in the context of their present health conditions, that the team collectively cannot as readily communicate. Therefore, practitioners carrying out one-to-one interventions can contribute significantly to team membership by relating their clients' life stories, thereby providing insights that promote effective teamwork, and, ultimately, positive treatment outcomes.

Repeated refrains from health and social service providers in teamwork workshops conducted at numerous health care facilities include: "teamwork is too time consuming," "teamwork doesn't lead to the best solutions," "the team leader takes over and we don't have an opportunity to state our views," "members of the team don't follow through on the decisions made at team meetings," "the physician doesn't show up or comes late," and "I might as well do all the work because I can only count on myself." It is evident that many teams are racked by tension and conflict that mitigate or, at worst, negate the value of teamwork. These attitudes are perhaps best expressed in the familiar quip, "What is a camel? A horse designed by a committee."

However, health and social service professionals, some in the early stages of their careers and others with many years of experience, admit that the teamwork workshop they are attending is often their first exposure to the art and science of teamwork These workshop participants, yearning to improve patients' quality of care, come to understand that effectively functioning interdisciplinary teams can:

- save time
- prevent duplication of efforts
- decrease fragmentation of care
- reduce single-perspective tunnel vision
- promote comprehensive care
- enhance coordination of care
- provide energy and synergy to team members

- increase patient collaboration, and
- improve quality of life for the older adults they serve (Leipzig et al., 2002; Miller & Toner, 1991; Siegler, Hyer, Fulmer, & Mezey, 1998; Toner, Miller, & Gurland, 1994).

## DEFINITIONS OF TEAMWORK

Historically, it was expected that the patient's physician would make most treatment decisions. Therefore, the work of a team of other health and social service professionals was limited. With advances in technology and greater opportunities for consumer education, patients themselves have become an integral part of the process, playing a critical role in their own treatment planning and decision making (Howe, Berglund, & Amato, 2000). In addition, the concept of teamwork has expanded with the decentralization or transfer of individual disciplines within a hospital to larger, multidisciplinary departments that are designed to function more efficiently. Also, the advent of managed care organizations and the need to compensate for scant resources currently encourage a team approach (Mellor, Hyer, & Howe, 2002). Therefore, if patient care and system-wide goals are to be achieved, health care and social service providers need to be much more conscious of defining their teams in both development and management phases.

"Many health professionals use the terms *multidisciplinary* and *interdisciplinary* interchangeably despite differences in the philosophy and practice of each" (Miller & Toner, 1991, p. 205). Members of multidisciplinary teams often work in the same organization, but frequently plan goals and interventions for their patients independently of other team members. Individual team members report, verbally or in writing, to the team as a whole with the aim of achieving coordinated care. "These pro forma meetings too often have a negative impact on decision-making since the outcome is compromised by failure to identify significant dynamic issues and examine alternatives" (Miller & Toner, 1991, p. 204).

In contrast, members of interdisciplinary teams assume joint responsibility for treatment outcomes by setting goals and making treatment decisions together. Collaboration among the team members, through formal and informal communication, is an explicit norm of interdisciplinary teams (Baldwin & Tsukuda, 1984; Campbell & Vivell, 1983; Miller & Toner, 1991).

The components of teamwork most consistent with this author's philosophy and practice are as follows:

- The interdisciplinary team is composed of a mix of professionals from various disciplines and are often employed by the same organization.
- Interdisciplinary team members share common goals, collaborate, and work interdependently in planning, problem solving, decision making, and evaluating team roles and functions.
- Team members, not only the designated leader, assume leadership roles to promote team objectives.
- Ongoing team discussions relate to interactional processes, such as developing and monitoring strategies for regular communication and defining and negotiating roles (Takamura, Bermost, & Stringfellow, 1979).

The immediate recipient of interdisciplinary teamwork is not always the individual patient. At times, informal caregivers (family members) or formal caregivers (home health aides, physicians), or the team itself (multiple disciplines in a health or social service agency) might be the direct beneficiaries of interdisciplinary teamwork, indirectly affecting the care and quality of life of the clients/patients they serve.

Two examples follow. If a family member is included in the team, she can describe her difficulties in caring for her relative. In one situation, a daughter's poor body mechanics in transferring her mother from bed to chair and on and off the toilet led to severe backaches. When she conveyed this information to the team, an occupational therapist was able to show her proper body mechanics in performing transfers that relieved her pain. In another situation, an elderly man complained to his social worker that his daughter was too nervous about having him leave his apartment by himself since he fell on the sidewalk, slipping on wet leaves. In a desire to help her father and keep him safe, the daughter was inadvertently fostering a sedentary lifestyle, thereby increasing his fall risk from prolonged inactivity. The social worker and therapists worked with the daughter and patient to encourage safe activity outside the home. This team discussion, with all the parties involved, increased the safe function and quality of life for this father, and his daughter was reassured that she did not have to worry about entertaining her dad all the time if he could get out to the senior center on his own.

## WORK GROUP DYNAMICS

Prior to receiving education in interdisciplinary teamwork, students and practitioners have been known to state, "We can't change the way our team works because we all have our own personalities" and/or "We can't buck the system; our organization has always been this way." One can't argue with the fact that we do have our own personalities and each system has requirements to fulfill that respond to local, state, and federal mandates. However, having a repertoire of conceptual frameworks to help understand the complex nature of individual and group behavior will provide team members and leaders with additional knowledge and skills to decrease the dysfunctional actions of teams and facilitate more functional, collaborative teamwork. Included are a few basic frameworks to ready students and practitioners for more effective team membership and leadership.

## General Systems Theory

Students and practitioners of health care are accustomed to thinking of the human body as a system with many subsystems (e.g., cardiopulmonary, digestive, musculoskeletal) that comprise the whole person. An example follows to illustrate the importance of General Systems Theory (GST) as a framework for providing quality care.

*A physician referred a patient to this author to improve function in his activities of everyday living. This 79-year-old gentleman, with osteoarthritis, emphysema, and diabetes, lived with his wife, who assisted him with most daily activities. Upon arrival, the occupational therapist observed a devoted wife and an alert, friendly, overweight man who was unable to transfer from bed to chair without assistance, considerable pain, shortness of breath, and dizziness. Before the evaluation was completed, the patient's wife offered the therapist and her husband homemade cookies. This man's excessive weight could not have helped any of his three conditions stated above. Another part of the system, then, outside the human body, was the patient's wife, who inadvertently affected her husband's health and ability to function, exacerbating signs and symptoms of distress. The patient's therapist needed to focus not only on the patient, but on his wife as well. How could she assist her to be helpful to her husband in a constructive way?*

This example illustrates how each subsystem and element within a larger system can either facilitate or impede function. If we take this example a step further, we can see how other elements in the larger system may affect outcomes for this patient. How does the financial status of this family affect the availability and frequency of services? Can they afford to receive therapy for as long as indicated and can they purchase needed medications? Will the landlord permit installation of bathroom grab bars to increase safety? Are other professionals indicated to facilitate an improved state of health?

A systems approach goes beyond the organ, to the individual, to family, community, and society. In addition, this small team (patient, wife, therapist, physician), each one a member of the larger system, can either be part of the problem or part of the solution. The very concept of system suggests elements that are related to each other and facilitate or constrain functioning. Functioning effectively depends on a variety of factors: (1) the individual members who are elements within it, (2) the relationship of the team to other professionals and to other teams, and (3) the equilibrium of the institution of which it is a part, all of which comprise the larger system. Through GST, practitioners can understand the behavior of humans and organizational behavior as well, which is the beginning of identifying problems accurately, choosing valid strategies for intervention, and solving problems more effectively and efficiently (Baum & Christiansen, 1997; Sampson & Marthas, 1990).

## Establishing Explicit Team Norms

All teams have norms that are expectations of behavior that individuals have toward each other and the group as a whole. These norms, some implicit and others explicit, influence the extent to which a team is functional or dysfunctional. Procedures and roles develop early, whereas values and commitment of the team evolve more slowly (Drinka & Clark, 2000). It may be implicit within a particular team, for example, that disagreement means unhealthy conflict, silence means agreement, and that certain members of the team can come late or not show up to team meetings without consequences (Miller, 1989; Rubin, Plovnick, & Fry, 1975). "Groupthink [Janis, 1972] refers to the tendency within many groups to eschew conflict and adopt a normative pattern in which the good group member is loyal to the group's leader and other members, never really challenging the leader's or the group's wisdom in matters of decision-making" (Sampson & Marthas, 1990, p. 79). Such implicit norms lead to highly dysfunctional teams.

If team norms are made explicit, especially in the development phase, many problems are obviated. For example, disagreement can be explicitly identified as healthy creative tension, based on mutual respect and an understanding that varied perspectives can lead to solutions of complex problems. If each team member, not only those with the highest status in a hierarchical structure, is recognized as contributing to the team's primary goal of achieving quality care, then more active involvement of all members who have contact with and knowledge about patients' needs and wishes will participate. Making team norms explicit reduces resentment engendered by a member's feeling superfluous to the team, decreases passive-aggressive behavior, such as saying "yes" to an action decided upon for a patient and then not following through, and enhances the interest of health and social service professionals in contributing to and attending team meetings (Miller, 1989; Miller & Toner, 1991; Sampson & Marthas, 1990; Toner et al., 1994).

## DEVELOPMENTAL STAGES OF TEAMS

The work of several social scientists (Bales, 1950; Bennis & Shepard, 1956; Bion, 1959; Sampson & Marthas, 1990; Tuckman, 1965) is especially useful in elucidating the issues that confront all teams and understanding the developmental sequence that teams experience. Issues of orientation, belonging, inclusion, and dependency often dominate the first stage of a work group's development. Typically, in the second stage are interpersonal issues, such as control, storming and fight/flight propensities that can be interrelated. Illustrations of these behaviors follow. Control issues have to do with membership and authority issues. Who is in charge? Who is most respected and listened to by the designated leader? Sometimes members vie for influence and status in the group. Leaders and members can assist each other by listening to each member's contributions and define and negotiate roles to the satisfaction of all involved, consistent with the mission of the team. Storming has to do with the arguments (fight behavior) that sometimes occur on teams impeding effective team functioning, i.e., collaborative work. Flight refers to escape behavior such as not listening to what is being said by someone on the team, digressing from the task at hand with a topic that is unrelated, coming late to meetings or not being present, physically and/or mentally. This occurs when individuals feel they do not belong, their contributions are not appreciated, and/or the goals and tasks of the work group are not clear and/or not valued by group members. However, it is important for team members and team leaders to recognize that some disagreement on a team is important in order to achieve creative solutions to complex problems. It takes mutual trust and respect for disagreements to occur leading to positive outcomes. When a team has weathered some of these struggles and moves on to function more effectively, a third stage is frequently characterized by norming. This developmental stage refers to teams that have successfully completed the prior stages of work group development with the result of mutual respect and affection. Performing, the last stage of team development, occurs when ongoing collaboration of a mature work group is ongoing (Sampson & Marthas, 1990).

Well-functioning teams do not often follow this sequence in a straight line, but rather a spiral, in which they move back and forth among these developmental stages and psychodynamic states. There are numerous reasons a group might deviate from following a developmental sequence. Examples include the facts that new members of a work group may not have been oriented fully to the team's mission, policies, and procedures; goals and roles may not have been adequately defined and/ or negotiated; explicit norms related to how to work collaboratively may not have been established; and the team may have been adversely affected by the presence of an authoritarian or laissez-faire leader.

Regardless of the theoretical framework, central to all work groups are issues of authority, leadership, and member-to-member relationships that need to be addressed before the team can function successfully (Sampson & Marthas, 1990). Becoming knowledgeable about work group dynamics enhances team members' abilities to diagnose problematic aspects of team functioning and intervene appropriately. The constraints of this chapter permit only a brief overview of these concepts.

## TEAM DEVELOPMENT

Team development includes, but is not limited to

- establishing clear, mutually agreed-upon goals,
- clarifying norms
- defining and negotiating roles
- developing membership/leadership guidelines
- learning to communicate (formally and informally) to promote collaboration and accountability.

First to be discussed are role definition and role negotiation, aspects of team development that are too often ignored on teams and are a frequent source of conflict. Leadership concepts will follow in order to increase readers' awareness that members can be leaders and leaders can be followers on a well-functioning interdisciplinary team.

## ROLE DEFINITION AND ROLE NEGOTIATION

When we hear words such as mother, pharmacist, nurse, teacher, or physician, we think of typical characteristics and functions that define these roles in society. Roles are positions that carry with them expectations of specific actions and responsibilities. Regardless of the individuals who occupy these roles, the standard expectations of behavior can become problematic when individuals do not fulfill their roles in the manner anticipated by team members or authority figures. Examples follow that describe the ways in which interdisciplinary teams can be more or less effective, depending on whether the roles of specific individuals on a team are understood by those with whom they collaborate.

In one nursing home, a new member of the team, an occupational therapist, expected to work closely with the nursing staff and dietician in order to maximize patients' abilities to feed themselves with minimal assistance from others. This would involve having the nursing staff make a list of the names of patients with difficulties in eye-hand coordination and/or limited motion and strength in one or both upper extremities. This list would then be used by the occupational therapist to assess patients with these limitations to determine if self-feeding using adaptive equipment, such as a built-up eating utensil, would enable individuals with limited grasp to function independently at mealtimes. Upon evaluation, the occupational therapist would then notify the dietician that adaptive equipment would be needed on the meal trays of particular patients for each meal. This appeared to be an excellent idea for facilitating maximum independence at mealtime, but when the occupational therapist told the nurses and dietician of her plan, she received a reserved "okay" response from the nurses and an "I'm not sure this will work" reply from the dietician. After two months of trying to implement the plan, it proved unworkable. Disappointed and angry, the occupational therapist wondered why the nurses and dietician, members of the same team, did not work with her to improve patient care.

Upon examination, the nurses and dietician concluded that this request was not part of their roles. This was "extra work" for staff members already feeling overburdened. The occupational therapist made assumptions about team member roles that were faulty. At a previous nursing home where the occupational therapist had worked, this self-feeding program was in place when she arrived. She assumed that nurses and dieticians fulfilled these tasks as part of their roles.

Although certain aspects of roles are indisputable, such as administering of medication by nurses, other elements of care need to be defined by the given team in a particular system and agreed upon by all the parties involved. Lack of clear communication fosters faulty assumptions and leads to role ambiguity, role overload, and passive or active resistance. Role clarification can occur when members take time to describe their roles and expectations to each other (Miller et al., 2001).

On a well-functioning interdisciplinary team, role definition and role negotiation (modifying roles) are ongoing as new members and new programs are introduced. Respect for individual differences of members is a norm of the team. Not all social workers, for example, have the same strengths, interests, preferences, and values. After professionals complete their education, they work in different types of facilities. One facility may be a general hospital where discharge planning and placement are the primary roles of social workers. At another facility, mental health counseling, that may or may not include discharge planning, may be their primary role. Other social workers might have developed personal interests through on-the-job training or continuing education, such as guided imagery, and wish to impart these skills to their clients in a new setting. These professionals will bring their added expertise and experience to new positions.

When teams take the time to learn the talents, limitations, and preferences of colleagues, they can achieve their goals more effectively, and the teams and the clients/patients they serve can be enriched. At the same time, achieving the mission of the organization as effectively and efficiently as possible must be the primary goal of the team. Therefore, role definition and role negotiation are ongoing processes.

## LEADERSHIP AND INTERDISCIPLINARY TEAMS

"What qualities do you hope to see in a leader of a team in which you are a member?" This question is frequently asked of health and social service professionals in courses and workshops on interdisciplinary teamwork. The qualities most wanted in a leader include being knowledgeable, competent, open, flexible, a visionary, accountable to others, trustworthy, charismatic, skillful at delegating, a good listener, a builder of alliances, and an advocate. When the participants are asked whether all of these qualities are frequently seen in the same person, they uniformly respond, "No." However, they all concur that these qualities are necessary for a team to be successful.

With the realization that any one person would have to be superhuman to have all the above-mentioned leadership qualities, an interdisciplinary team recognizes that members can and should assert leadership behaviors. Leaders with self-awareness, who recognize their preferences and limitations in leadership styles, should delegate leadership responsibilities to other members of the team when situations warrant it (Toner et al., 1994).

The work of R. F. Bales (1950, 1970) is particularly useful in assisting team members and designated team leaders to recognize the two kinds of behavior needed on teams in order to accomplish goals effectively and efficiently. Bales (1950) describes task behavior, which helps the group fulfill the mission of the agency and the goals of the particular team, and socioemotional or maintenance behavior, which has to do with the interpersonal relations on a team related to keeping the team running smoothly (e.g., communicating effectively and demonstrating respect for members' opinions).

Knowledge of task roles and group maintenance roles can be used to foster positive leadership behavior for all members of the team and to monitor individual members' and team performance. Examples of helpful task behavior include seeking information, giving opinions, clarifying, elaborating, and summarizing. Maintenance behavior includes encouraging, harmonizing, compromising, facilitating communication, and setting standards and goals for the group. Designated team leaders and team members need to monitor themselves continually in order to achieve a balance between task and maintenance behavior. Some teams are task focused to the extent that the needs of members are overlooked, whereas other teams overemphasize "feeling good," resulting in less effective and efficient teamwork.

Baldwin and Tsukuda (1984, p. 428) describe the "emerging norm on many primary care teams, which appears to be one of equal participation and responsibility on the part of team members." Interdisciplinary teams are encouraged to make the norm of rotating and sharing leadership functions explicit and to avoid placing all hopes in one leader (e.g., the charismatic leader), who may foster dependency and/or leave the team to fend for itself at some point in time (Toner et al., 1994).

A democratic leadership style is the approach of choice on interdisciplinary and multidisciplinary teams. The ultimate clinical decision maker may remain the physician, but a nurse, occupational therapist, or social worker might be the formal team leader, as that person's particular skills might be indicated for a particular situation (Drinka & Clark, 2000). Crisis situations are an exception to democratic leadership; the imminent need for intervention calls for authoritarian leadership (Miller & Toner, 1991). The study of leadership styles in health care organizations, as they specifically affect outcomes of client/patient care, remains a relatively untapped and potentially important area of research.

## TEAM MANAGEMENT

When goals for the interdisciplinary team have been established in the context of the mission of the organization, specifically the needs of the older adults being served, and norms are made explicit, roles have been defined and negotiated, and a system for leading and communicating are clear, then the team is ready to move from team development to team management. It is important to remember that because of the nature of teams (i.e., some members leaving, new members joining, policies and procedures changing, programs being added, modified, and/or replaced) development remains ongoing within the management phase of interdisciplinary teamwork (Miller et al., 2001).

Team management, like team development, is also client-centered. This might seem obvious, but sometimes members of a team can get caught up in the status and power of the "work group" and inadvertently assume they know what is best for clients, omitting clients themselves, who are also team members, in the process of critical decision making about their health and their lives. To achieve optimal care and quality of life for the older adults we serve, clients and their families need to be included in treatment planning and decision making whenever feasible.

Effective management on an interdisciplinary team signifies that an ongoing, comprehensive, and coordinated system for evaluation and intervention with older adults exists to improve their health and quality of life. Communicating verbally and in writing about patient care and using a system that can be monitored to evaluate the extent to which explicit goals are being met are essential components of team management. Team members from different disciplines contribute to the comprehensive evaluation process by conducting formal, standardized assessments of cognitive, physical, psychological, and social functioning and/or by giving and receiving informal information about the lifestyle, habits, needs, interests, and wishes of specific patients. The outcomes of these evaluations are discussed at team meetings, sometimes called case conferences.

## SYSTEMATIC PROBLEM-SOLVING (SPS)

"Systematic Problem-Solving" (SPS), a six-step problem-solving process, was developed as a team management strategy to identify and solve complex patient problems and system-wide problems that affect the quality of patient care (Miller & Toner, 1991). Since the initial development of SPS, the author and J. A. Toner consulted at several mental health institutions, teaching SPS to newly forming and ongoing teams.

For more than a decade, through the New York-Geriatric Education Centers Consortium, instruction in SPS has been provided several times a year to practitioners throughout New York State. Participants choose problems that they are currently experiencing in their work settings, and bring back creative, doable solutions that arise from the SPS process to their own facilities for consideration and possible implementation. The six-step process, followed by an example, is outlined below (Miller, 1993).

## Step 1 (Defining the Problem)

"A problem exists when a goal is unreachable or if there is a discrepancy between the way things are and the way things ought to be" (Center for Interdisciplinary Education in Allied Health, 1980, p. 116). To define the problem accurately, it is necessary to ask as many questions as possible. Questions that begin with who, when, and where are useful in eliciting facts; questions that begin with what, how, or why are likely to be most effective in stimulating thinking about solutions.

## Step 2 (Brainstorming Solutions)

Brainstorming, as defined in this process, involves generating one idea from each participant while postponing any judgment as to its efficacy. Any suggestions regarding ways to solve the identified problem are encouraged by the facilitator without criticism or premature rejection. Members who prefer not to take a turn or whose idea was already stated can say "pass." In this way, each member has an opportunity to speak, but does not feel coerced.

## Step 3 (Choosing a Solution)

All ideas generated in the brainstorming session are reviewed and the possible solutions are discussed. The merits of each solution are evaluated in terms of three criteria: time, cost, and enthusiasm of the participants. The choice of solutions is arrived at by group consensus.

## Step 4 (Planning Ways to Implement the Solution(s)

Delegation of responsibilities for carrying out one or more of the solutions is essential before acting. Roles are defined and negotiated, and commitments and tasks that members will undertake are recorded.

## Step 5 (Carrying Out the Plan)

An appropriate time to carry out the plan is established, and the suggestions developed in steps 3 and 4 are put into practice. It should be noted that difficulties that impede progress toward a solution often arise when the plan is being carried out. In that case, members meet again to evaluate them.

## Step 6 (Evaluating the Solution)

"Within an agreed-upon time, it is determined whether the plan of action is working. If it is not completely satisfactory to any one person involved and if modifications are indicated, the problem-solving steps are reintroduced. Ongoing support from administration is vital to success" (Miller & Toner, 1991, pp. 211–212).

### *The Case of Mr. J.*

*Mr. J. is a 76-year-old man with diagnoses of paranoid schizophrenia, diabetes, and mental retardation (MR) (IQ = 84) and a past history of violent behavior and post-operative cataract surgery. The staff requested that SPS be applied to Mr. J.'s care, with J. A. Toner and the author as facilitators, because the patient had numerous problems that seemed intransigent. The presenting physical problems were dermatitis and self-inflicted bruises. Behavioral problems included stuffing toilets with soap and towels, urinating in inappropriate places (shoes and drinking fountain), stealing other people's food, eating too fast and sometimes choking, and hoarding items stolen from other patients. After discussion, the staff came up with the following plan.*

## Step 1 (Problem Definition)

How might we relieve skin and behavioral problems of Mr. J. to improve medical and psychosocial conditions?

## Step 2 (Brainstorming Solutions)

The following possible solutions were generated: (1) Send Mr. J. to the bathroom right after meals to avoid urinating in shoes. (2) Tell Mr. J.

not to urinate in the drinking fountain, and then if he does he will have to wash the fountain. (3) Use repetition and frequent directions because of MR. (4) Provide psychological testing to determine current cognitive status. (5) Use positive reinforcement for appropriate behavior. (6) Give Mr. J. jobs to do to occupy him, provide feelings of usefulness, and reduce aggression. (7) Engage him in an exercise program. (8) Assess range of motion and strength because of complaints of pain in his shoulders. (9) Remind Mr. J. not to scratch himself. (10) Use Benadryl to promote sleep and reduce nighttime disruptive behavior. (11) Apply skin medication twice instead of once a day.

## Steps 3 & 4 (Choosing Solutions and Planning Methods to Implement Them)

These activities led to the following plans: (1) Nursing staff will be consistent and get Mr. J. on a regular bathroom schedule. (2) All disciplines will give Mr. J. directions more frequently. (3) A social worker will notify psychology about psychological testing. (4) An occupational therapist will evaluate his physical condition and encourage him to participate in an exercise program. (5) A recreation therapist will give Mr. J. jobs to do, such as washing the dining room tables. (6) Nurses and other disciplines will frequently remind Mr. J. not to scratch. (7) Nurses and other disciplines will give Mr. J. rewards for appropriate behavior, such as diet soda and ice water (team reminded by nursing of his diabetes). (8) Staff will postpone giving Benadryl until other strategies have been tried. (9) Nurses will consult with the physician if skin condition persists after behavioral interventions are tried.

## Steps 5 and 6 (Implement Solutions and Evaluate Their Effectiveness)

These steps could not be observed by the facilitators, as they were visiting consultants to the institution. However, reports immediately after the meeting were positive. Members of the team stated that they were very glad they took the time to have an SPS team meeting about Mr. J. They reported "improved morale," on realizing that they had options available to improve Mr. J.'s medical and psychosocial conditions that they had not considered, and most important, they reported "being pleased that they could learn from each other in this format."

SPS, part of team management, enables application of "best practice" procedures in a systematic way. A collaborative process, with all team members participating, is encouraged, providing a sense of ownership to all involved. The process of SPS is task focused in that members share information, initiating, clarifying, stating opinions, recording results, and summarizing.

## Team Process

On a well-functioning team, members are concerned not only with what is said or not said, but why. It is understood that both verbal and nonverbal behavior can influence the productivity of the team, thereby ultimately affecting patient care. Team process discussions are a way for teams to monitor their own performance in a structured, supportive environment (Miller, 1989). A team leader or team member at the end of a meeting can ask the team, "Have we achieved our goals for the day? How did we do? What can we do better?" It takes secure members, with explicit norms, to continue to improve team functioning by addressing these questions. The author models this behavior by asking these questions of her patients and her students. The process of SPS, a structured, safe format, also fosters team maintenance behavior, as members and leaders learn to disagree constructively, thereby reducing or avoiding resentment, passive-aggressive behavior, and premature and inaccurate decision making.

## CONCLUSION

If the multiple, complex needs of older adults are to be met, interdisciplinary teamwork is essential. The sooner students and practitioners learn to work collaboratively and interdependently, the more likely comprehensive and coordinated care will be available to the increasing percentage of individuals living to advanced ages. Teamwork can be learned. It is an art and a science that includes understanding and applying the three elements of teamwork: team development, team management, and team process in the context of work group dynamics. Health care and social service practitioners have a desire and responsibility to provide quality care. It is hoped that this introduction to interdisciplinary teamwork will help team members to work more effectively.

# REFERENCES

Baldwin, D., & Tsukuda, R. (1984). Interdisciplinary teams. In C. Cassell & J. Walsh (Eds.), *Geriatric medicine: Medical, psychiatric and pharmacological topics, Vol. 2* (pp. 421–435). New York: Springer.

Bales, R. F. (1950). A set of categories for the analysis of small group interaction. *American Sociological Review, 15,* 257–263.

Bales, R. F. (1970). *Personality and interpersonal behavior.* New York: Holt, Rinehart & Winston.

Baum, C., & Christiansen, C. (1997). The occupational therapy context: Philosophy—principles—practice. *Occupational therapy: Enabling function and well-being* (2nd ed., pp. 26–45). Thorofare, NJ: Slack.

Bennis, W. B., & Shepard, H. A. (1956). A theory of group development. *Human Relations, 9,* 415–438.

Bion, W. R. (1959). *Experiences in groups.* New York: Basic Books.

Campbell, L., & Vivell, S. (1983). *Interdisciplinary team training for primary care in geriatrics: An educational model for program development and evaluation.* Los Angeles: Veterans Administration Medical Center.

Center for Interdisciplinary Education in Allied Health. (1980). *Health systems* (Clerkship study guide and resource manual). Lexington, KY: University of Kentucky Press.

Drinka, T. J. K., & Clark, P. G. (2000). *Health care teamwork: Interdisciplinary practice and teaching.* Westport, CT: Auburn House.

Howe, J., Berglund, K., & Amato, N. (2000). *Mount Sinai geriatric interdisciplinary team training manual.* The Mount Sinai GITT Program, The Henry L. Schwartz Department of Geriatrics and Adult Development & Bronx VA GRECC Program, New York.

Janis, I. (1972). *Victims of groupthink.* Boston, MA: Houghton Mifflin.

Leipzig, R. M., Hyer, K., Ek., K., Wallenstein, S., Vezina, M. L., Fairchild, S., Cassell, C. K., & Howe, J. L. (2002). Attitudes toward working on interdisciplinary healthcare teams: A comparison by discipline. *Journal of the American Geriatrics Society, 50,* 1141–1148.

Mellor, M. J., Hyer, K., & Howe, J. L. (2002). The geriatric interdisciplinary team approach: Challenges and opportunities in educating trainees together from a variety of disciplines. *Educational Gerontology, 28,* 867–880.

Miller, P. A. (1989). Teaching process: Its importance in geriatric teamwork. *Physical and Occupational Therapy in Geriatrics, 6*(3/4), 121–131.

Miller, P. A. (1993). Problem-solving in long-term care: A systematic approach to promoting adaptive behavior. In J. Toner, L. M. Tepper, & B. Greenfield (Eds.), *Long-term care: Management, scope and practical issues* (pp. 107–122). Philadelphia: Charles.

Miller, P. A., Hedden, J., Argento, L., Vaccarro, M., Murad, V., & Dionne, W. (2001). A team approach to health promotion of community elders. *Journal of Occupational Therapy in Health Care, 14*(3/4), 17–34.

Miller, P. A., & Toner, J. A. (1991). The making of a geriatric team. In W. Myers (Ed.), *New techniques in the psychotherapy of older patients* (pp. 203–219). Baltimore, MD: American Psychiatric Press.

Rubin, I., Plovnick, M., & Fry, R. (1975). *Improving the coordination of care: A program for health team development.* Cambridge, MA: Ballinger.

Sampson, E. E., & Marthas, M. (1990). *Group process for the health professions* (3rd ed.). Albany, NY: Delmar.

Siegler, E. L., Hyer, K., Fulmer, T., & Mezey, M. (Eds.). (1998). *Geriatric interdisciplinary team training.* New York: Springer.

Takamura, J., Bermost, L., & Stringfellow, L. (1979). *Health team development.* Honolulu, HI: University of Hawaii, John A. Burns School of Medicine.

Toner, J. A., Miller, P. A., & Gurland, B. J. (1994). Conceptual, theoretical, and practical approaches to the development of interdisciplinary teams: A transactional model. *Educational Gerontology, 20,* 53–69.

Tuckman, B. W. (1965). Developmental sequence in small groups. *Psychological Bulletin, 63,* 384–399.

# Appendix 1

# Sample Bereavement Support Letter to Families of Deceased Hospice Clients

HOSPICE OF KERSHAW COUNTY
KERSHAW COUNTY MEDICAL CENTER

Date: _____

Dear (client's family),

On behalf of Hospice of Kershaw County, we would like to extend our deepest sympathy in regard to your loss. We are honored to have had the opportunity to help in providing care for your loved one. As a result, our lives have been touched and enriched.

Our staff was touched with your loving care, and the grief you may be feeling now. As the days, weeks and months go by, please remember that we are still here for you. If you would like to talk about your loved one and your loss, or if there is anything you are concerned about, please give us a call. We would be pleased to hear from you.

In the meantime, we hope the enclosed information on the grief process will be helpful to you and your family. We have also enclosed a form for our assessment of your need for bereavement support from Hospice. We will contact you shortly to help you complete this form—either over the phone or in person. You can stop by our office, or we can come to your home. This assessment gives you the opportunity to let us know how we can best serve you. We hope that you will help us to help you.

Sincerely,

_____     _____     _____
(signature)              (signature)              (signature)
Family Support           Bereavement              Volunteer
Counselor                Coordinator

# Appendix 2

## Bereavement Assessment Form

HOSPICE BEREAVEMENT ASSESSMENT
TO THE ATTENTION OF BEREAVEMENT CLIENTS

Dear Friends: The purpose of this form is to help you to understand your grief experience. While grief is a universal experience, grieving is a very individual process, which each person experiences in his or her own way. For example, there is no set timetable or best technique for coping with the loss of a loved one. However, if the pain of your grief seems unbearable or overwhelming without relief, and/or if you feel out of control and helpless much of the time, we want to help you. You may talk freely with our Hospice bereavement staff, including our volunteer chaplains and other counselors. We all are available and ready to comfort you and to help you understand what you are going through. Understanding your grief makes it easier to handle.

We urge you to take a little time to use this form to assess the impact of your loss by identifying problems that are getting in the way of your healing process. Enclosed is a stamped envelope for the return of this form. When we receive it, we will call you to arrange for whatever bereavement support your assessment indicates that you may need. A note about confidentiality: Please be assured that any and all information gathered by Hospice for the purpose of evaluating your service needs and providing bereavement support to you is confidential and may be shared with others only as approved by you and as necessary in order to plan and provide assistance.

(1.) General Information
Your name and address _____
Your phone number (   ) _____
Your loved one's name _____
Date and location of his/her death _____

## (2.) Support
Do you have family, friends or concerned others who are available to you with whom you can talk about the pain of your loss? ____ yes, or ____ no. If "no", please tell us more.

## (3.) Employment
Are you experiencing difficulties at work that you think may be due to your loss? ____ yes, or ____ no, or ____ not applicable. If "yes," tell us more.

## (4.) Your Physical Status
Are you having any of the following problems continually? Check those which pertain to you: ____ I can't sleep, ____ I sleep too much, ____ I have no appetite, ____ I eat too much, ____ I don't pay attention to my appearance, ____ I've gained a lot of weight, ____ I've lost a lot of weight. Tell us about any physical reactions to your loss that worry you (e.g., sense of emptiness or hollowness inside, tightness in your chest or throat, shortness of breath, weakness in your limbs, no energy, dry mouth and others):

## (5.) Your Feelings
Grieving persons may experience many emotions ranging from love to anger, frustration, numbness, anxiety, guilt and others. Do any of these common feelings or others seem to be of unusual intensity or more than you can bear? ____ no, ____ yes, ____ sometimes. If you checked "yes," or "sometimes," tell us more.

## (6.) Worrisome Behaviors & Thoughts
You may be concerned about certain of your behaviors or thoughts that you did not experience before your loss. Let us know what they are: ____ I act withdrawn, ____ I am very restless, never seem to be able to concentrate, ____ I act irritated too much of the time, ____ I have thought about suicide, ____ I drink too much alcohol (describe): ____ I am taking a lot of pills, or other drugs (describe): ____

## (7.) Stresses
Are you having difficulties in the following areas that may be adding to your feeling of loss and hindering your healing process? ____ finances, ____ your living situation, ____ your health, ____ other problems. Please tell us more. We want to help.

(8.) Other Problems
Please check here if you would rather identify these stresses over the
phone or in person. Is there anything else not covered so far that you
think may be interfering with your healing process? If so, let us know.
Perhaps we can help _____
____ Please check here if you would rather tell us over the phone, or
in person

(9.) Please sign this form.
Your signature: _____
Date: _____

(10.) Bereavement Follow-up
Signature & title of Hospice assessor _____

Plan/intervention: follows: ____ no follow-up is required or recommended, or care plan as follows:

_____

_____

# Index

Edentulism, 150
Education, 10
EEOC, 226–227
Elder abuse, 245–256
  aggressive patient, 250–251
  caregiver risks, 250
  elder costs, 252–253
  false accusations, 252
  family caregivers, 251–252
  investigating, 248–249
  reporting, 248–252, 249
  untrained caregivers, 253
  written abuse, 249–250
Elder costs
  elder abuse, 252–253
Elder fraud, 253–256
Elderly
  approach to, 120–121
  atypical disease presentation, 119
  diseases specific to, 118–124
  frail
    home health care, 9
  law, 217–227
  nonspecific disease presentation,
    119–120
Emotional abuse, 246
Employee Retirement and Income Se-
    curity Act (ERISA), 227
Employees
  environmental gerontology, 65
  nursing home
    innovative empowerment models,
    52
  recruiting and retaining
    nursing homes, 49–52
End-of-life issues
  Alzheimer's disease, 191–193
  cultural competency, 194
  differentiation, 190–191
  economic factors, 187–188
  feelings, 195–196
  social service perspective, 185–199
Endurance
  environmental design, 70
Environmental change
  case study, 74
Environmental design, 63–80
  agility, 70
  Alzheimer's disease, 70–71
  benchmarks, 80
  communication barriers, 70
  detractors, 70

direct caregivers, 75–77
endurance, 70
nursing homes transformation,
    73–75
Environmental gerontology
  assisted independence, 64
  concerns, 64–66
  design implications, 68
  functional design, 65
  functional independence, 64
  theoretical progress, 66–68
Equal Employment Opportunity Com-
    mission (EEOC), 226–227
ERISA, 227
Estate planning, 222
Ethical dilemmas, 231–232
Ethics, 229–244
  defined, 230
  institutional settings, 235–237
  social issues, 234–235
  society, 243
Ethnic composition, 9–10
Ethnic woman, 35
Exercise, 128, 134
Expenditures
  out-of-pocket, 19

Failure to thrive, 119
Falls, 116–117
Familiar stimuli, 72
Family, 54
  changes, 26
  dementia, 37–38
  historical perspectives, 26–27
  reservoir of wisdom, 29
  therapeutic intervention, 177–179
  traditional values, 26
Family caregivers, 35–37, 177
  elder abuse, 251–252
Family relationships, 25–38
Family traditions
  transmission, 29
Fat, 130–131
Federal funding
  aging programs, 55
  HCBS, 55
Feelings
  about parents, 27–28
  communicating, 28
  end-of-life issues, 195–196
  positive, 27–28
Financial concerns, 117

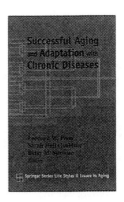

Lightning Source UK Ltd.
Milton Keynes UK
30 January 2011

166620UK00001B/11/A

9 780826 125750